Surviving the Pink Ribbon

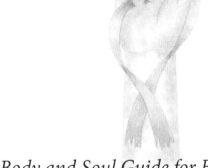

Body and Soul Guide for Breast Cancer Survivors and Co-Survivors

Rita Schunk

Live Learn
LOVE
Publishing, LLC

This book is designed to provide helpful information. It has been written in good faith and is accurate to the best of the author's knowledge. The information presented is not intended as medical advice and may not be advisable to your situation. Appropriate health care professionals must be consulted to tailor any changes to your specific needs. The publisher, author, and all parties involved in the development of this book disclaim all liability related to the use of this book. Therefore, they are not liable for any damage or negative results from any treatment, action, or application to any person reading or following the information contained within. Readers should be aware that the websites listed in this book may change.

Scripture quotations are from the World English Bible version (Public domain)

Copyright © 2018 by Rita Schunk
Live Learn Love Publishing, LLC
Mount Horeb, Wisconsin
ISBN: 978-1-7324193-0-8
Library of Congress Control number: 2018909445

Cover design by Christine Keleny ◆ ckbookspublishing.com
Cover image by Rhonda Saylor Wolf
Author photo by Brittany Johnson ◆ Reverie-Photography.com
For information or to contact author, go to
www.RitaSchunk.wordpress.com

Dedicated to:

∽

My late-husband, John, who taught me
how to live courageously

My husband, Jim, who believes in me

My son, Eric, who is the best part of me

Contents

Foreword ∼

Surviving the Pink Ribbon: Body and Soul Guide for Breast Cancer Survivors and Co-Survivors ticks all the right boxes. Rita Schunk's ability to foreground often overlooked details helps readers to understand *why* they are essential.

Because breast cancer does not discriminate, the author penned this book for women of every age and walk of life, and those who love them. Understanding the correlation between positivity and the success of treatment, the information in this book is uplifting while at the same time, realistic—and often humorous:

"'Demo' surgeon? I now refer to Dr. D as my "demo" surgeon because I think of the mastectomy in kitchen remodeling terms. Dr. D will do demolition work, then the plastic surgeon will build the new "cabinets". While

the lymph node core biopsy is scheduled,
I visit with a plastic surgeon to learn about
"cabinet" building and picking out a "knob"
style."

I wish *Surviving the Pink Ribbon* had been available when my mother had breast cancer resulting in a radical mastectomy. The experiential wisdom in the "Helpful Strands" section at the end of each chapter contains actionable suggestions for survivors (one becomes a survivor on the day of a cancer diagnosis) and co-survivors (the people who love them). They're full of great advice like, "Once the plan is known, create a countdown tool for the survivor. One example: a paper chain with one link for each chemo treatment. Write an encouraging thought on each link for the survivor to read and break off after each session."

Rita goes on to say, "Cancer treatment is not a sprint, it's a marathon. Get your body and soul ready. Spend the necessary time along the way to take care of all of you." This book is designed to help readers take a holistic approach—body, mind, and spirit.

Surviving the Pink Ribbon: Body and Soul Guide for Breast Cancer Survivors and Co-Survivors is an uplifting companion, support, and resource tool. Rita is realistic, relevant, and honest: "Does all this freak me out? Yup!"

As a holistic health practitioner, I've learned that not everyone is looking for an answer. Often, people just want to be heard. Rita shares that "The best gift to give is the gift of presence. Be available to listen to the survivor. You do not need to offer solutions."

The suggestions woven throughout this book come from hard-won experience. They're not only practical; they're achievable. Here are but two examples:

- Have a dentist appointment right before you begin chemo. You won't be able to see a dentist while you are in chemo treatment.
- Wipes are more comfortable than toilet paper when you have no hair down there.

In the spirit of being active rather than passive, Rita shares that "Planning and proactive action provide an illusion of some control." One of the many applaudable action steps that she took—I love her warrior attitude—is detailed in this brief excerpt:

"The oncology nurse mentioned yesterday that my hair will start to fall out in a week and will be entirely gone a week after that. So, I've decided to lose my hair on my own terms. Next week I have an appointment with the salon to get my head shaved. In preparation, I pick up some soft cotton yarn to knit myself a bedtime cap."

Rita is not only a survivor, she is also a thriver. The sharing of her experiences in the pages of *Surviving the Pink Ribbon* will help others to do the same.

—LAURIE BUCHANAN, PHD, holistic health practitioner, transformational life coach, keynote speaker, and award-winning author of *Note to Self: A Seven-Step Path to Gratitude and Growth*, and *The Business of Being: Soul Purpose In and Out of the Workplace.*

Preface ～

"This will be my last blog post. Thank you for stalking me and posting comments. You were critical to my mental health as you encouraged me, challenged me, and made me laugh so hard I cried. Still, I'm looking forward to having a life that is not so interesting."

The final blog entry done. With breast cancer now in the rear-view mirror, I'm not looking back. Or so I thought.

I could ignore the pushing from family and friends. The internal nagging was too insistent. *What about the women being diagnosed with breast cancer every day? What about their friends and family? How many times did you hear "let me know how I can help"? Now you know how to answer. Remember how many times during this journey you felt as if you were the first person to have breast cancer? You can prevent others from feeling that way. You have answers to getting through this more comfortably. Don't keep them to yourself.*

I've long believed life's experiences are not to be wasted. They are to be learned from and shared, especially/even when the tuition is paid in fear, confusion, and pain. I had paid tuition again and again through diagnosis, treatment planning, chemotherapy, surgery, and radiation. I had wished for an experienced friend to come alongside me, someone who could give me answers – not for medical questions – but for how to make it through. How to care for my body and soul as they were repeatedly assaulted.

And I heard "let me know how I can help" from well-meaning family and friends – my co-survivors. I wish I had a nickel for every time I heard that platitude. In the heat of my cancer battle, I usually did not know what help I needed. Now I do. So, I decided to document one path through breast cancer, my path. My fears. My confusion. My learning processes. What helped me. This includes some honest (and not so reverent) words to my Heavenly Father and some words from the book he wrote to me (the Bible). Whether or not you have a relationship with God, I hope these words bring perspective and comfort.

- If you have been diagnosed with breast cancer (a survivor so far), this book is your experienced friend.

- If you know someone with breast cancer, this book is your guide as a co-survivor.

- If you are wondering what day-to-day life is like for a person with breast cancer, this book will help you understand.

I wrote this for you. I had to.

Introduction 〜

Pink has always been my favorite color. But it takes more than pink ribbons to get through breast cancer. While a knowledgeable medical team and appropriate medical treatments are critical, I'm convinced that comfort for the body and soul is vital as well. The state of your body and soul can affect treatment success.

Medicine is constantly changing and is unique to each person. This book focuses rather on the body and soul impacts during a breast cancer journey. Each chapter walks you along a path through breast cancer. My experiences as I moved through diagnosis, treatment planning, chemotherapy, targeted therapy, surgery, and radiation are covered. At the end of each chapter are Helpful Strands of advice as to how to keep your body and soul more prepared and comfortable during that part of the journey.

Friends and family of a person with breast cancer, the survivor, will see themselves as each chapter unfolds. These co-survivors also have Helpful Strands to grasp at each chapter's end. The chapter on support is a place for co-survivors to reflect on their relationship with the survivor.

Another place of reflection is in the final chapter. Whether you are a survivor, a co-survivor, or are just wondering how someone could say, like I have, that cancer was a blessing in disguise, you will find the answers here.

～ 1 ～

DIAGNOSIS
Say the Words

The phone rings. I stop typing on the computer to squint at the caller id. It's the doctor's office – the call I've been expecting. I glance at my watch – exactly four p.m. I take a deep breath and answer the phone with the automatic, company-policy greeting I always use.

The nurse gets to the point quickly. We have met just once, but she knows me well enough to understand that I appreciate the direct, no-nonsense approach. As she starts talking, however, I think, *I'm not ready. Maybe this should wait until my doctor's appointment tomorrow*. Too late. She reports that I have breast cancer. I grab a scrap of paper and a

1

pen. I've cared for others enough to know I won't remember anything she says next. Her words are as unfamiliar as background conversation in a foreign land. I strain—confused for a moment.

"Please repeat the name of the cancer and spell it for me," I ask.

"I…N…V…A…S…I…V…E…D…U…C… T…A…L…C…A…R…C…I…N…O…M…A. Invasive ductal carcinoma". I'm reduced to a recording machine as I take in letters and copy them down.

3 centimeters… grade 3… most aggressive… lots of ductal carcinoma in situ, I write.

The conversation is brief. I hang up the phone. Just half an hour more to work, but that's too long. I shut down my computer, grab my purse, and head for the exit.

Please don't let me run into anyone; I can't say words right now. Please keep me alive long enough to get home; I can't breathe. Please get the traffic out of the way for me; I am driving in a seriously impaired state. Home is 18 miles away past acres of green crops and occasional simple farm buildings. *Didn't I pass that barn already?* I am afraid to take a breath, afraid of what may happen if I do. So, I swallow air in tiny erratic sips.

2

I pull up to our house, slam the car into park, and sprint toward my husband. He sees me and switches off the lawnmower.

"I have breast cancer," I blurt out using my last bit of breath.

I fall into his arms, finally able to find a breath – just enough to cry. And, as I say the words and tell my husband the news, I find I am also telling myself.

❦ Two weeks ago ❧

After my regular mammogram, the clinic asks me to return for another look at my left breast. *Why can't they squeeze it harder the first time, so I don't have to come back?* I return to Medical Imaging at the clinic, more than a little annoyed, but the young female technician is so nice I can't stay bothered. She takes a few pictures of the left breast.

"I get my clothes back on now and you'll call me if there is something interesting, right?" I turn to follow her out.

"No, please keep the robe on, and wait in this room. The radiologist will look at this right now," she replies, and closes the door behind her.

The service is never this good, even when I've returned in the past. Maybe they're trying out a new process. Or maybe there's a problem. Maybe cancer. No, that wouldn't make sense. I focus on the room. Sofa, coffee table, magazines. Nice little living room. I perch on the edge of the sofa – uncomfortable on this comfy couch. I stroke the terrycloth robe. *It will be OK, right God?*

In just a few minutes, the door opens and in walks the technician along with a young male radiologist. He reviewed the test and compared it to last year's. He offers to contact my regular doctor at once to facilitate the scheduling of a visit with a surgeon to biopsy my left breast. Surgeons have worked on a large benign cyst on my left ovary, a calcium deposit in my left rotator cuff muscle, and a hernia on the left side of my groin – now my left breast. What is it with the left side of my body?

The radiologist speaks with my regular doctor and an appointment is set up with a surgeon before I leave. This is Thursday. The following Monday my husband and I meet with the surgeon to discuss what type of breast biopsy would best diagnose the problem. At this point, I am still hopeful that it may be some weird lump and not cancer. That is, until the surgeon explains that a five on the BI-RADS scale is highly suggestive of malignancy. And the radiologist rated the spot on the mammogram at a five. When I go home and look up the scale on a reliable source on the internet, a "five" in a study is cancerous in 95-97% of cases. I feel as if my last hope to avoid a cancer diagnosis is likely gone.

The surgeon explains biopsy options and we agree on an ultrasound-guided needle biopsy in my case. The procedure is scheduled for a week and a half later. This is way too far in the future for my comfort, but it is the soonest available. I fill the time by going to work each day, harvesting vegetables from our garden, and keeping up with errands. I get my hair trimmed – must look nice for the procedure. And I find the perfect shoes for my son's upcoming wedding. The wedding is over a year away, but I aspired to find good-looking and comfortable shoes. I don't have a dress yet, but these shoes will work with anything. Spoiler alert: cancer treatment makes sure that I will never wear these shoes.

Breast biopsy day comes. The procedure is scheduled for early afternoon, we sleep in and try to relax. The typical surgery prep is done. Time to wheel me in on the gurney. "You're going to put me under, right?" They say they are not, which I take as a joke. They aren't kidding. They don't put me under – just give me medication to relax and make me not care so much. Another thing that helps is that my husband, Jim, is allowed to stay in the room. There is quite the crowd around my "girls". The right one is being pushed out of the way, while the left breast has an ultrasound "mouse" driven across. The doctor moves what looks like a #8 knitting needle in and out and around inside the breast. This is all quite unpleasant and a bit uncomfortable, but the procedure seems over quickly. They leave a titanium clip where they remove the tissue as a sort of bookmark. Whether or not this turns out as a cancerous tumor, future medical staff will see the clip and know that this suspicious spot has already been biopsied. Then I have a mammogram done on this now sore breast to ensure the clip is in place and all is done. I feel quite bruised, but I feel able to go to work the next day. And that next day is Thursday, the day I receive the "cancer" call. But hearing "cancer" is not the same as saying the words myself.

❦ ❦

But cancer! I am the middle child in a family of nine – five sisters and three brothers. None of us has ever been afflicted with cancer. I don't even know anyone who has cancer! I'm the vegetarian who has never smoked, gave birth when young (in my twenties), and breast fed my son for three months.

There is no reason for me to get breast cancer. Then again, there's no reason for me not to. Instead of "why me?", how about "why not me?"

One of my next thoughts is to somehow tell my son, Eric. He's living 100+ miles away and is engaged to be married. Saying the words to my husband hurt, and I don't believe I can get the words out to my son. I'm sure I will start to sob after the first word. So, my husband offers to call Eric at work. Eric works second shift in a hospital lab. Jim is Eric's stepfather. Eric's dad died during Eric's high school years. After the news, Eric steps to the other side of the lab and took a "moment" to compose himself. Eric and I are somewhat conditioned to medical issues by my late husband's extensive history of life-threatening conditions. But this time, I'm the one needing care.

Soon after phoning my son, a sister calls. "Let's visit mom all together and take an informal family photo tonight. I know this is last-minute, but you can come, right?" My siblings and I live in southern Wisconsin, except for a sister in Florida and a brother in Texas. The planets have aligned—all nine of us are near the Madison nursing home that my mom is calling home. A family party is the last thing I want to do. I have received a life-changing, life-threatening diagnosis a couple of hours ago. I need time.

"I'm too tired from work. I don't feel well," I reply. That isn't like me. I always show up to family get-togethers. These excuses are lame. I have no brain power to spare to make up better ones. Since the cancer news, my mind is a car in need of a tune-up – full speed ahead with intermittent backfires. Progress in gathering information and creating a list of questions with sudden brief thoughts of "Is this real? How could this happen?" I skip to the last stage of grief—acceptance. Then I flip back to the first stage—denial.

My sister counters every excuse. "This won't take long." "How often are all of us together?" "I'll come and pick you up." And the ultimate – "Do this for mom."

I look at Jim – my face pleading. *Help me figure out how to get out of this!* But his face is simply supportive. He knows that I know the right thing to do. And so, I do.

Jim and I arrive at the nursing home. I'm wearing a black shirt to match my mood. I do not want family around with these medical words swirling in my head. I can't make small talk and smile for the photo. But I do. Jim does a lot of the talking for me and stays by my side. My plan is to spread the word that I have something to say, and to meet me in the parking lot after the visit with mom. If I feel I can do it, that is when I will inform my brothers and sisters of my diagnosis.

And that is how I tell them – standing in a circle in front of the nursing home. "About four hours ago, I learned that I have breast cancer." Surprised looks. My tears can no longer be held, and I see tears forming on faces around me. No one moves, so I go to them, hugging each in turn around the circle. My brothers are a bit stiff, not used to expressing love to their sister in that way.

"Well, I can't steal your toys to get your attention anymore, so as the middle child I have to come up with a different way," I joke. "I figure breast cancer will do it." To my surprise, I am wrong about that (as you'll see in the chapter on Support).

Now it's Thursday evening. This afternoon I received the news that I have cancer. Analyzing and organizing is what I do at work. I'm an IT project manager. I need to treat this cancer thing like a project. I need to find out everything I can about this type of breast cancer and write down questions for the appointment with the surgeon tomorrow. My first stops are the American Cancer Society website (www.cancer.org) and the Susan G. Komen website (ww5.Komen.org). The sites provide some basic information and questions to take to my doctor. Good thing they have lists of questions I can use, because right now I don't even know what to ask. Well, I guess there is one question that overrides all the thoughts swirling in my head: *How do I get this cancer out of my body?* I need the doctor to answer this at my appointment tomorrow morning.

Helpful Strands ~
Diagnosis

Survivor

- Information can help, confuse, and scare. Gather enough information from reputable sources to feel empowered. But don't search and consume to the point of being overwhelmed. I set a limit as to how much time I would spend on this, and how many sources I would use. Information is necessary, but a clear head is too.

- These are some of the websites I found helpful: www.BreastCancer.org, www. Cancer.org (American Cancer Society), www.Cancer.gov (National Cancer Institute), www.MayoClinic.org (Mayo Clinic), www. MDAnderson.org (MD Anderson Cancer Center), and ww5.Komen.org (Susan G.

Komen). Also, Gilda's Club or another affiliate of the Cancer Support Community (www.CancerSupportCommunity.org) will have a cancer-focused library and helpful people. I am fortunate to have a Gilda's Club close to my home. Gilda's Club is a non-profit organization providing support to anyone touched by cancer.

- Get copies of each test result. I found myself referring to these while researching to understand what applied to my situation and what did not.

- As needed, ask the medical team to speak slowly and repeat. The brain can only process so fast.

- Ask the medical team to answer important questions as soon as possible or direct you to a person or place where the answer may be found. Not knowing is more difficult than whatever the answer may be.

- My mind often felt like a computer screen with too many windows open. None of the windows were minimized. And new windows were opening faster than I could deal with. Persist and move forward knowing this feeling will pass. Ask for help to deal with and close windows.

- Decide which thing is the most urgent or is most bothersome. Focus on that, and get it dealt with and settled as much as possible. Then move onto another. Take one step at a time, or even just one moment at a time.

- I slipped into the "why me?" moments. But I got to thinking that maybe the question is not "why me?", but "why not me?". Why should I be more fortunate than so many others? Maybe God will use this to mold and shape my character, stretch me, give me experiences I should use to help others. Stay open to what can be learned through this journey. Do not waste this experience.

- Fear and faith cannot occupy the same space. Fear can be a sign of doubt in God and His plan. When scary feelings arrive, be reminded that feelings come and go, but faith endures. Focus on who God is and what He has done. Let faith push fear out of the way. The Book of Philippians contains many passages to help cope with anxiety.

- Do a "trust fall" into God's arms. Settle into His support. As Psalms 46:10-11 states: "Be still, and know that I am God... Yahweh of Armies is with us. The God of Jacob is our refuge." Matthew 11:28 states: "Come to me, all you who labor and are heavily burdened, and I will give you rest." 1 Peter 5:7 states: "casting all your worries on Him, because He cares for you."

- Sometimes I tried to put God on hold – too consumed to focus on God, to understand what He may doing, or even to pray. God can't be paused. And that's good. Remember that God is merely a thought away. He's always there – right there – and He wants to abide with you. As Hebrews 4:15-16 states: "For we don't have a high priest who can't be touched with the feeling of our infirmities, but one who has in all points tempted like we are, yet without sin. Let's therefore draw near with boldness to the throne of grace, that we may receive mercy and may find grace for help in time of need."

Co-survivors

- Offer to drive the survivor to appointments and procedures. Offer to wait in the waiting room. Knowing that a welcoming face will be greeting you can make a person's day. If you are close enough to the survivor, taking notes during the appointment can be helpful.

- The best gift to give is the gift of presence. Be available to listen to the survivor. You do not need to offer solutions.

- Search for a "window" you can help close. The survivor may not know what she needs right now. So simply offer something you can do. Offer to make calls, pick something up, bring food from the survivor's favorite take-out place, clean the house or a room or a countertop, etc.

- When you're with the survivor, keep tissues handy. Her emotions may be all over the map, and she may not be prepared. And you may need them too. Sometimes having a good cry together is just what's needed.

- Avoid adding any complexity to the survivor's life. Don't ask her to choose the restaurant, suggest one. Don't ask which day and time to do something, suggest a day and time. Help either to make or to avoid non-critical decisions right now.

- Send an encouraging note or card. A funny card that has nothing to do with cancer can be much needed comic relief.

- Take care of yourself. As they say on airplanes, "Put your oxygen mask on first before you help someone with theirs." Also, Galatians 6 mentions to bear your burden, then bear one another's.

- Ask the medical team to recommend good sources of information. Suggest the survivor limit the amount of time gathering information so as to not become overwhelmed or confused.

~ 2 ~

TREATMENT PLAN
Arm Yourself

I feel nervous, but prepared, as Jim and I sit in the surgeon's office. My homework is done. In a notebook, I copied the few facts about my breast cancer diagnosis his nurse stated on the phone yesterday. To that I added 15 questions I saw on the cancer websites I visited last night. I left two lines after each question to write in the surgeon's answers. This preparation and organization is giving me the slight bit of control I need to hang onto at this moment. I cling tightly to this notebook. Since the phone call yesterday, this notebook has become my lifeline.

Dr. D enters and takes a seat next to me at

the desk. He likes the fact that I am prepared with questions. He's going to go through the breast biopsy results in more detail and describe treatment options. He expects that he will answer my questions as he does this, but I am welcome to ask any unanswered ones at the end. *Good, he's got this* – another small measure of comfort – my grip on the notebook releases a bit. He asks if he can borrow my notebook. He wants to write notes for me as he speaks, so my husband and I can focus on what he is saying. I am immediately thankful for wherever he learned this method of communication. I take a deep breath and reluctantly hand over the notebook.

Dr. D flips through the pages until he finds a blank one. He sketches pictures as he describes the anatomy of the breast, milk ducts, and what the cancer cells have been busy doing while I lived my life. He carefully writes the long, technical words as he explains them. Then he outlines the three-step plan to deal with the cancer: surgery, chemotherapy, and radiation. He talks about the surgery options first: lumpectomy (removal of part of the breast) or mastectomy (complete removal of the breast). He diagrams where some lymph nodes are in relation to my left breast and talks about testing the node under my arm closest to the tumor during the surgery. If the lymph node tests positive for cancer, most of the lymph nodes in my armpit will also be removed during the surgery. He mentions chemotherapy as a possible follow-up to surgery. Radiation is only mentioned as something done with a lumpectomy.

As far as timing goes, he suggests that I see a breast reconstruction surgeon he usually works with next week, because the beginnings of that process can take place at the same time as the breast surgery. I would be off work for about two weeks after the surgery, then chemo would start a week or so after that. I would likely have chemo for six months – one session every three to four weeks. From start to finish, the plan will take seven months. That seems like a long time, but if that's what it takes to get rid of this cancer, let's do it – and get started now!

Dr. D reminds me there is time to think things through. I'll get a second opinion, and he encourages that. But suddenly, I am aware of the alien presence in my body that I want to get rid of now! There is a "large mass" in my breast, "lots" of ductal carcinoma in situ (DCIS) all over that same breast. DCIS are pre-cancer cells in the breast ducts that have not formed a tumor yet. And the pathology reveals this invasive ductal carcinoma forming the "large mass" also is, in my case, the most aggressive strain. I want to have the surgery as soon as possible and start the process of removing and attacking these wayward cells. My historically well-functioning body has turned on me. I don't drink, I don't smoke, and I'm a vegetarian. Yet I now have cancer.

Next step. Just focus on the next step. I call the clinic to arrange for copies of the mammograms, the notes, and the biopsy pathology report. I get a copy for myself and learn that sending these straight from the clinic to the doctor is the fastest method of communication. OK, now I need to select a doctor for a second opinion. Right away I decide that I want to select someone outside of my health plan – I want a fresh opinion – and I want this done soon.

First, calls to some of my sisters for surgeon names. A general surgeon's name is suggested, but no one I know has cancer experience. I'm thinking I need more of a specialist. Next, a famous clinic that has a lot of specialists. I could see a breast specialist in a week, then meet with some surgeon two weeks after that. *No, three weeks is too long. I don't have any idea where this cancer may have gotten to in my body already. I can't wait that long.* On to a "cancer" hospital. Even though they work with many kinds of insurance, they don't work with mine (*of course*). I could be seen next week (*great!*), I would visit for three days (*OK, I guess*), and I would have to give them an enormous deposit (*no way!*). Moving on to a local hospital. It takes many phone calls to various departments, but I now have an appointment for next week with a breast surgeon, Dr. B. Another mammogram will be done beforehand. My insurance won't cover this, but we will get the money together. It's a plan.

Although I have a plan to proceed for my body, there's no plan for helping my mind through this. I decide that my energies will focus on getting rid of the cancer. So, I begin paperwork for absence from work for the entire course of my treatment – whatever that may be. After a month, I will be on short-term disability. That will be 60% of my pay, minus some taxes, and minus my health insurance premium. I decide to refinance my mortgage to be able to live on reduced funds.

Speaking of caring for my mind, how will I communicate with eight brothers and sisters and numerous friends during this treatment process? I'll go crazy doing it via email and phone. And I'm not on social media. While on the hospital's website, I see a link to www.carepages.com. It's super easy to set up your own page through them. Only the people you invite may see your page. I will be able to post updates and photos, and my invitees can view them and post comments. CarePages becomes a communications and sanity lifesaver.

I have a plan for my body and my mind. How about my spirit? My spirit has been tested and fortified over many years. I believe my spirit is ready. The testing has come through being a caregiver to my late husband. We were together almost 20 years. He was completely blind by the time we started dating. A kidney transplant, quintuple heart bypass, life-threatening infections, congestive heart failure, and multiple amputations followed – all from the ravages of Type 1 diabetes. Don't get me wrong. There were wonderfully amazing times in between. And, through it all, we leaned on God and each other. God turned these experiences into character-building education that worked as mortar to build each of us personally and cemented us together. I believe everything that comes into my life is there for a reason. And cancer is no exception. God plans experiences to build my character and make me better able to fulfill the purposes He has for me. Give God control of the situation. After all, he has held control all along. This is happening *for* me, not *to* me. Through the grace and strength from my relationship with God, I clung to these promises within hours of getting that phone call with the diagnosis. Jim and I are at the start of this journey through breast cancer, and I already see signs that God's hand is doing the same through this experience.

Waiting a week for the second opinion is difficult. Work, Jim's presence, and preparing for my body and soul to join in the fight help the time pass. The tests and meeting with the second opinion surgeon were much like the first round. However, one big plan-altering revelation surfaced. Dr. B. recommends a lymph node core biopsy be done now. She says if the results are negative, I should proceed as planned (surgery, then chemo, then perhaps radiation). However, if the results are positive, scans should be done to look for where the cancer may have spread. And I would likely want to do chemo before surgery. This makes a lot of sense to me. It satisfies my "attack everywhere – all at once" urges. I don't know why Dr. D didn't mention this possibility. Through countless phone calls and being quite pushy, I am able to get my "demo" surgeon to discuss approaches with Dr. B. They both agree to move forward with a lymph node core biopsy. My "demo" surgeon's nurse says it will be at least a couple of weeks before the biopsy can happen. After some pushing, the procedure is set for late the following week. I will be at the hospital most of the day. This is a more complex procedure than the breast biopsy. I decide not to ask if I will be awake for this one as I'd rather be surprised. Being awake for the other biopsy was lots of fun! Or not.

"Demo" surgeon? I now refer to Dr. D as my "demo" surgeon because I think of the mastectomy in kitchen remodeling terms. Dr. D will do demolition work, then the plastic surgeon will build the new "cabinets". While the lymph node core biopsy is scheduled, I visit with a plastic surgeon to learn about "cabinet" building and picking out a "knob" style. In my case, the "remodeling" process will take a year. I will have a large scar on the back of my shoulder, must take an antibiotic before any future dental work, have several additional drains after the mastectomy surgery, and must change out the implant every 10 years. Yikes! I decide to investigate the breast prosthesis option. There are many realistic-looking and -feeling options. But what about mastectomy bras?

The sole place my insurance will cover mastectomy bras is through a company that sells durable medical equipment (wheelchairs, walkers, crutches, etc.). In my quest to fully research the prosthesis option, I decide to check it out. Jim and I meet the mastectomy specialist in a small office with a desk, computer and metal cabinet. The specialist looks about my mom's age (mid-80s), but I figure that means she is experienced. I take off everything from my waist up – something I seem to do each time I have an appointment nowadays. She measures me and asks if I want to try on the most popular bra. Sure! She reaches into the cabinet and brings out a bulky corset-looking bra with a wide clasp containing four or five hooks. I obediently try it on. Yes, all my pieces and parts are securely kept in place as she promises. But this looks like something even my mom wouldn't wear. Maybe my grandmother would, if she were still alive. After the appointment we are disheartened. After going to the websites of the companies she works with, I find many mastectomy bras that look just like the functional, but pretty, bras I currently wear. At least they exist.

Something else happens during this week before the next biopsy. Jim gifts me with some expensive chocolate for now (I heard a comedienne once say that chocolate helps fluff breasts up after a mammogram – and mine have been through a lot in recent weeks!) and a bag of individually wrapped chocolates for later, when I need a little something. He also gives me two enormous binders, because he noticed I already filled up a small binder with papers from doctors and research. He read in *Breast Cancer Husband* by Marc Silver (a book the surgeon recommended) that women can stuff a three-inch binder. He wanted to make sure I have what I need. He also purchases pretty flowered dividers and some clear page sleeves. Perfect. And he gives me a book, *After Breast Cancer: A Common-Sense Guide to Life After Treatment* by Hester Hill Schnipper, LICSW, to encourage me to look forward. He's such an amazing guy! There is so much information and so many aspects to breast cancer. I am taking time today to better organize myself. I decide to read just one book right now, *Dr. Susan Love's Breast Book* by Susan M. Love, MD, to avoid further information overload. Reading helps me understand, but it also raises my anxiety level. I move my mind back and am thankful for what I have and what I can count on – back to prayer – staying connected to God.

Now it's time for the lymph node core biopsy. The process is comparable to the breast biopsy, but with more prep and more "digging". Jim convinces them to let him stay in the room during the procedure. As a retired cop, he's seen a lot, but they make him sit in a chair just in case. They can't have the distraction of a fainting husband. They give me drugs through the IV that relax me but still allow me to answer their questions. The process takes longer than the previous biopsy and is more painful, but still manageable. Jim says they took at least 10 samples from two lymph nodes. What I know is there is a lot of hard pushing around the area under my left arm for those apparently elusive nodes while someone else on my right slides the ultrasound "mouse" around the same area to guide the search. Highly uncomfortable in so many ways. I am told to ice the area and avoid pushing or lifting for five days. We should have the results in a day or two.

The next day I decide to work from home. The area feels puffy and bruised. And I've developed some type of nerve issue. When I move my left arm a certain way, I have a pain that shoots up my arm. I feel a bit mentally bruised too. I am waiting for a result to direct me to surgery or chemo as soon as I can arrange it. I want to be home for this call. The day ends and there is no call. I feel as though we are on the cusp of being able to start fighting back against this cancer. Well, maybe tomorrow.

Tomorrow is Friday the 13th of July—three weeks since my diagnosis. This is not a lucky day for me. The "demo" surgeon tells us that the breast cancer has travelled to my axillary (armpit) lymph nodes. Both nodes tested positive for cancer. At least now we know. The "demo" surgeon will contact the oncologist he recommends to get an appointment next week. He already sent two other women for their first oncology visit, so he isn't sure how soon they can see me. But we do know the first step: chemotherapy, not surgery, because the immediate concern is preventing the cancer from progressing further. It's time to start fighting back!

Helpful Strands ∾
Treatment Planning

Survivor

- Once you have garnered test results, opinions, and options and have a plan for treatment, take comfort in being ready to fight back. Don't spend time second-guessing and considering the what-ifs. Be confident that your plan suits you. Don't compare your plan to someone else's or their outcome. Guard your mind and spirit by avoiding people who want to compare their plan or that of someone they know. Each body, breast cancer, and treatment combination is unique. Yours is best for you.

- Stay open to the possibility of change along the way. And know that, although you may be taken by surprise, God is not. As Proverbs 16:9 states: "A man's heart plans his course, but Yahweh directs his steps."

- A cancer treatment plan consists of many components, and there is much to consider when creating your plan. Keep good notes. Take someone along to your appointments – both of you taking notes and comparing later.

- Ask the medical staff to write some notes, print test results, and print helpful information. This allows focus on the conversation and provides items that can be referenced later.

- Ask the medical staff to make specific commitments and keep them. Ask them who specifically is available to answer questions and how they can be reached.

- Push to keep moving forward or have someone advocate for you. The polite, but firm, squeaky wheel does get the grease (or whatever is needed) sooner.

- Find an easy way to keep family and friends up to date. I found that establishing a Care Page saved me time in keeping my co-survivors informed. Encouraging comments they posted were a bonus. Caring Bridge (www. CaringBridge.org) has similar functionality to CarePages, which unfortunately no longer exists. And I am sure there are others.

- You may know the cancer's stage. Or you may

never know. People will ask. If the cancer cannot be staged, get an answer ready. My response in general involves a short statement about the fact that, because of the order of my treatments, the cancer could not be staged.

- Cancer treatment is not a sprint, it's a marathon. Get your body and soul ready. Spend the necessary time along the way to take care of all of you.

- Be sure to include fun activities and rewards in the treatment plan. Something to look forward to. Just be prepared to cancel, if your health doesn't allow for the event.

- When I feel inadequate and overwhelmed, I am comforted in knowing that God is in control, and that the Holy Spirit will interpret and communicate my needs to God even when I can't. Romans 8:26-28 reminds me: "In the same way, the Spirit also helps our weaknesses, for we don't know how to pray as we ought. But the Spirit himself makes intercession for us with groanings which can't be uttered. He who searches the hearts knows what is on the Spirit's mind, because he makes intercession for the saints according to God. We know that all things work together for good for those who love God, for those who are called according to his purpose."

- When I pray for patience during a time of frustration, I seem to wind up in traffic jams and long lines at the store. I guess I am gifted with many opportunities to practice the patience I am desiring. James 1:2-4 states: "Count it all joy, my brothers, when you fall into various temptations, knowing that the testing of your faith produces endurance. Let endurance have its perfect work, that you may be perfect and complete, lacking in nothing."

Co-survivors

- Volunteer to attend the survivor's appointments. Give the survivor choices: drive them, accompany them into the appointment and take notes, or just sit in the waiting room to keep them company. Sometimes simply your presence can be invaluable.
- Keep communication flowing. Send cards to the survivor. Listen to the survivor. Being heard and validated is so important.
- Lift the survivor's spirits by doing something

for her. Not sure what to do? What do you imagine you would like? What are you good at doing? Do that. Don't let lack of knowledge or indecision paralyze you. Almost anything is better than nothing. Keep up the normal activities you do if her schedule and condition allow.

- Once the plan is known, create a countdown tool for the survivor. One example: a paper chain with one link for each chemo treatment. Write an encouraging thought on each link for the survivor to read and break off after each session.
- Arrange a fundraiser to help with medical expenses.

~ 3 ~

CHEMOTHERAPY AND OTHER DRUGS
The Fight Is On!

My son, Eric, makes the 100-mile trip to my first visit with the oncologist. As the nurse leads Jim, Eric, and me to Dr. A's office, we chat about music. The nurse refers to Jim and Eric as my backup singers. We have a laugh at the thought of the guys making coordinated dance moves alongside me. After introductions, Dr. A takes a blank sheet of paper and starts making diagrams and notes as he talks. I love that. He first summarizes the pathology aspects of my version of breast cancer. He assures me there is a known and effective set of drugs to administer. He is quite optimistic in a realistic sort of way. It is at once clear that he is treating us – Eric, Jim, and me. Although I am the primary person in this fight, I can tell that he believes their roles are also critical. They must be mentally and physically ready too.

Cancer is a condition where cells keep growing out of control, whereas they should grow, do their work, and then die off naturally. My version of breast cancer is progesterone receptor negative (cancer cells that do not feed on progesterone), estrogen receptor weakly positive (1% of my cancer cells feed on estrogen), and Her-2/neu positive (I have too many copies of an oncogene that tells cells to grow). I have either Stage II or III cancer. It is impossible to say, as the solitary way to stage the cancer is by having surgery, and I won't be having surgery until after some drugs have already done their work.

A term Dr. A is using a lot is neoadjuvant. Neoadjuvant describes the treatment approach we're using. In a neoadjuvant approach, therapeutic agents are administered before the main treatment. In my case, these are chemo drugs before mastectomy surgery. The drugs will all be administered through an IV, as opposed to some drugs that are oral. The summary of the plan is AC-TH. I'll receive Adriamycin and Cyclophosphamide once every three weeks for a total of four treatments (they call them "cycles"). Then I will receive Taxol every week for a total of 12 treatments. At the same time as Taxol, I will start receiving Herceptin. Herceptin is not a chemo drug. It is a targeted therapy drug. It is an antibody that blocks Her-2/neu. After I finish the six months of chemo, the application of Herceptin will be reduced from weekly to once every three weeks until I have a year's worth of Herceptin. So, I will be receiving Herceptin while I have surgery and radiation. We are throwing all options at this cancer since it has already travelled from my breast to the lymphatic system. This seems like a lot of medication and coordination, but I am wholly on board with putting up a major fight against these crazy cells in my body – taking the fight to wherever they may be.

Before we start, I have an echocardiogram to make sure my heart is in good shape. Herceptin can negatively affect the heart muscle, so we need a baseline and to know my heart is starting from a good place. Blood tests are also done to get a baseline to make sure there is no suggestion of any other issues. Since I will be getting drugs often through an IV over the course of 15 months, a port will be implanted into my chest. Because I want to begin the treatment as soon as I can, there is not enough time to get the port procedure done. The first chemo treatment is planned for a week from today using an IV in my arm. Early the next morning following the first treatment, I will get the port implanted just beneath my skin for the administration of the drugs and for the frequent monitoring of blood levels. Jim and I ask about doing some type of body scan to see where the cancer may be, if anywhere else. Dr. A says it is not necessary. The scan may show possibilities which we would then need more tests to track down – costing time and worry. And, in the end, the treatment will be no different. We are already planning to hit this with all that medical science has to offer. Jim and I must agree with that logic. But concern about not having a body scan will continue to surface from time to time throughout my treatment. Dr. A patiently explains each time Jim or I bring it up.

We meet with one of the chemo nurses. She shows us a port—a tiny purple alien space ship with three sides each about one and a half inches long. The nurse also gives us many documents – several describing the port, others describing the medications used to prevent or at least minimize nausea and other adverse chemo drug reactions, and a page for each chemo drug listing side effects and special instructions to follow when receiving the drug. The drugs taken to prevent nausea and drug reactions also have side effects. The effects range from minor (headache and temporary taste changes, for example) to life-threatening heart failure. Side effects vary, but there are two that are certain for me, since the first two drugs I will receive are the nastiest. I will have nausea and I will lose all my hair – all over my body. The nurse explains that they are well equipped to prevent nausea. Their goal is to make sure I never vomit – not once. The plan is to administer anti-nausea drugs via IV before the chemo drugs, then follow up with an intense schedule of pills for three days after each chemo session. If that isn't enough, they can do more. Does all this freak me out? Yup!

This week before the first chemo session, Jim and I purchase supplies to make me comfortable and to manage the most common side effects. Planning and proactive action provide an illusion of some control. We buy over the counter meds for headache, constipation, diarrhea, etc. I contact the American Cancer Society to provide a wig, since my insurance will not pay for a "cranial hair prosthesis". I start the paperwork to begin a Family Medical Leave Act absence starting the day of my first chemo session. I fill the prescriptions for anti-nausea pills and lidocaine jelly. The lidocaine is spread on the skin over the port before I come in for each chemo session. It numbs the area a bit so connecting to the port is not as painful. Let me assure you that it is still painful, just not quite as much. I read each word of the 20 pages that the oncology nurse gave me. It's frightening stuff. I keep reminding myself that they are listing all possibilities – hopefully much of this information will turn out not to pertain to me. There are a lot of detailed and practical methods listed to deal with pain, fatigue, nausea, hydration, mouth and throat problems, nutrition, diarrhea, constipation, hair and skin changes, and sexuality issues. The papers mention health care power of attorney. I'm in good shape there. The papers also mention that I will not be able to see the dentist during chemo, so I make an appointment to get a checkup done as soon as possible. Well, I guess I am as prepared as I can be. The fight is on!

A package arrives from the American Cancer Society. It contains a couple of light fabric head covers made by volunteers in South Dakota and Iowa. What a nice surprise to receive the day before chemo starts. From what I've been told, all my hair will be gone by the second or third treatment. I review the scarf tying instructions I picked up in a waiting room. I look through the few scarves I own – looking for at least one 36-inch square or 36 inches by 14 inches. I don't have any that are suitable. Well, at least I have the two head covers from these volunteers. Maybe I will knit or sew some.

It's chemo day – at last! Jim, Eric, and I take the elevator to the fourth floor in the same office building where we met the oncologist. Before we see Dr. A, I have a chest x-ray, they get my vitals (temperature, blood pressure, and weight), and draw blood. I, and my backup singers, follow the nurse back to Dr. A's office. He does a physical exam, reviews the x-ray and blood results, then pronounces me fit and able to move forward to receive the first treatment. I'm pleased that there are no last-minute glitches. I've been so ready and anxious to start fighting back against this cancer, since the day of my diagnosis – now five weeks ago. We go back to the waiting area. I notice a wicker basket in the middle of a table. It is filled with hats and scarves made and donated by volunteers as gifts for the oncology patients. And I see a clear glass candy dish at the end of the receptionist's counter. I find out later that these are ginger candies to help deal with nausea. I'm nervous as to what receiving chemo will feel like and how my body will react. I have received much information, yet I still don't know what will happen in my situation. The nurse calls my name and the three of us follow through the door. We pass row after row of cubicles – as in an office – each beige cubicle containing a tan recliner upholstered with a vinyl-looking fabric.

At the end of the cubicle rows, we enter a large room to have privacy during this first treatment. Or is it because my backup singers and I look a bit rowdy? I settle into the recliner while Jim and Eric have a seat in simple chairs. Out the window is a corn field in the middle of this business park—a field of bright green. I provide my name and date of birth to the nurse, which will become known as my secret chemo password. The saline IV gets hooked up, and we begin the short wait while the chemo drugs are concocted. The pharmacy waits to do this until I show up and the doctor determines that I am well enough to receive treatment. Soon a clear plastic shoe-box is delivered overflowing with IV bags of clear fluid and two "turkey baster" plastic syringes full of bright red fluid. That's the nastiest drug. The nurse pulls on special protective gloves and takes a seat almost too close. She connects a "turkey baster" to the IV and pushes the plunger ever so slightly. She looks at her watch for a moment or two, then nudges the plunger again. This process repeats until both large syringes are empty. Since much fluid is being forced into me, I carefully take the IV pole several times with me to the bathroom. The nurse mentions the red drug may discolor my urine. What an understatement. Soon after the red drug is administered, I pee in neon pink. If I turn out the bathroom light, I'm sure my pink pee would glow. I come back to the treatment room laughing. My husband and son look worried that something has put me over the edge until I let them in on the pink pee. Other than that, treatment is thankfully uneventful.

During treatment, we have visitors. What a delightful surprise. A friend checks in on how the first treatment is going. The social worker for the clinic also comes by. She gives us a cookbook for cancer patients, *The Cancer Survival Cookbook* by Donna L. Weihofen, RD, MS, with Christina Marino, MD, MPH. Since it is the same as Jim already purchased, Eric takes this one home with him. He plans to make some of the recipes this weekend for our freezer.

After treatment, Eric reveals he has started a team for the September Susan G. Komen walk in Milwaukee. What an important and beautiful way to show support. Will I be well enough to travel to Milwaukee by then, much less walk? Eric heads to work while Jim and I have a light lunch. We stop by to visit with my mom at the nursing home. Based on the recommendations of her caregivers, I will not be telling mom that I have cancer. She has dementia. She will not remember and I would have to re-explain. She doesn't need extra worry to affect her health. When I lose my hair, I'll just wear a wig to visit. And, if I don't believe I can pull it off, I'll just have to skip visiting for a while. I hope it doesn't come to that. We arrive home and I'm still feeling good – or maybe it's the nervous adrenalin still in my system. I step on the treadmill for a walk while I have the energy. I get to sleep in tomorrow, because Dr. A has postponed implanting the port until three days before my next treatment. He wants it implanted closer to when it will be first used.

The day after the first treatment I have a hot flash and a mild headache. I take an afternoon nap. Otherwise things are OK thus far. The oncology nurse mentioned yesterday that my hair will start to fall out in a week and will be entirely gone a week after that. So, I've decided to lose my hair on my own terms. Next week I have an appointment with the salon to get my head shaved. In preparation, I pick up some soft cotton yarn to knit myself a bedtime cap. The nausea has been warded off by the three IV drugs at treatment and the rigorous schedule of two drugs I'm taking for the next few days. One challenge for me is to drink as much as they suggest, 80-90 ounces per day, without using our tap water. Since we have well water, they want me to use bottled water instead. I'm not used to drinking in such large quantities. I'm keeping up, but it's a challenge.

How many times have I said, "It's just hair. It'll grow back," at the salon when getting a trim. I've never been fussy about my hair, and I guess that's a good thing right now. Jim and Eric look on as my hair is buzzed to the lowest setting on the clippers. The oncology nurses advise me not to go any shorter, because of the possibility of scraping my scalp by accident and risking infection. The head shave is a surprisingly festive experience – lots of laughs and photos. I save a lock of my hair to compare when my hair returns. The woman at the salon helps me pick out the color and style for a wig from the American Cancer Society's TLC catalogue. I'm ambivalent about using a wig, but I'll have it for visiting my mom. And, since insurance won't pay for a "cranial hair prosthesis", the wig's cost will be for the most part covered by the American Cancer Society.

Today is my first day without anti-nausea medications. So far, so good. I am sipping liquids throughout the day and eating five to six small meals each day as that should help. Another thing I need to do right now is make sure I am eating plenty of fiber. To that end I make a batch of zucchini/oatmeal/ wheat muffins. Eric and his fiancée visit and deliver several homemade soups for the freezer. I'm OK cooking for now, but it's nice to have that backup. I'm walking and trying out yoga to keep my body in fighting form.

My wig arrives in the mail. The style is longer and thicker than my hair. And, unlike mine, the wig has no well-earned gray highlights. Jim and I head back to the salon where she trims the wig to more closely match my style. Now I'll be able to visit my mom again. I can always say that I colored my hair and am trying out a little different style in preparation for Eric's wedding next year.

Today is the day to get the port implanted. We arrive at the hospital at 6 a.m. for the typical pre-surgery process. At 8:30 a.m. I am wheeled into surgery. The procedure will take about one and a half hours. They advise me that I will be awake for the procedure – not cool! But they give me drugs so I won't remember the most interesting parts. They place the port under my skin just below my collar bone and above the top of my bra cup on my right side—the opposite side of the cancer. They also place a little "hose" under my skin connecting the port to the jugular vein on the right side of my neck.

I wonder how they do this, and afterward I'm glad I don't remember that part. I imagine, "Just a little nick in the jugular and we'll be good to go!". The process is both creepy and cool. I am wheeled back to my room to get the drugs out of my system before returning home. I'm sleepy but smiling – one more step in this marathon. I merely need Tylenol for pain. At home I notice my neck is blue – the color of the antiseptic they used. My fingers easily trace the tube running up the right side of my neck just under the skin, and I feel it move a little as I move my head. That's so weird. Speaking of my head, it is staying toasty warm thanks to a cap a friend knitted for me.

Here we are, three days after the port implant, which is still bruised and swollen, and it's time for the next session of chemo. There are five of us today: one of my sisters, two friends, Jim, and me. After making sure that I'm still "vital", I get blood drawn through the port for the first time. It's a bit painful because of the tenderness from the surgery, but it works fine. Dr. A looks at the blood levels and comments that they have recovered to their pre-chemo levels. They won't be able to do that after further treatments, but it's a good way to start. Dr. A also does a physical exam. Jim and I are shocked to hear him say that the tumor is already less defined. He would now describe the tumor as a suspicious thickening if someone came to him for the first time. This is clear evidence that these first two drugs are having the desired impact – and after just one session! Jim and I break into happy, grateful tears at this news. The nurse reunites us with our posse and leads us to the treatment side of the clinic. We walk past the cubicles to a room with actual walls and a door. We affectionately call this the party room. They connect the next set of drugs to the port. The administering of the drugs is a bit quicker now – still takes hours though – since the jugular vein is a bigger "pipe" than what's in my arm.

The process repeats. The fight is on!

Helpful Strands ~
Chemotherapy

Survivor

- Treatment should reduce chance of recurrence, but it is not possible to get the recurrence possibility to zero. That is a big scary truth I came to terms with. But, hey, there are many things that have just as slim a chance of happening to me. And I don't go around worrying about them.

- Have a dentist appointment right before you begin chemo. You won't be able to see a dentist while you are in chemo treatment.

- Ask the medical staff to explain terminology and be ready to re-explain. This is a lot to take in.

- Visit www.ChemoExperts.com. This site provides information on cancer drugs and their side effects in three formats: reading, listening, and watching video.

- Ask the medical staff to be aware of your co-survivors, how they are doing, and what they may need. If the medical team is good at their job, this will happen naturally. Co-survivors need compliments and encouragement too.

- I am the same with or without hair. Maybe a bit funnier without hair. Wear a wig, wear a scarf or hat, or go with whatever is going on with your hair at the time – whatever works for you in the moment.

- Look for weird and funny things during treatment. I promise you they exist. Laughter helps.

- Remember that you are never alone. Matthew 28:20 states: "… I am with you always, even to the end of the age. Amen." Psalms 121:8 states: "Yahweh will keep your going out and your coming in, from this time forward, and forever more." And Psalms 121:4 states: "Behold, he who keeps Israel will neither slumber nor sleep."

Co-survivors

- The gift of presence is priceless. My co-survivors and I told stories and laughed through the hours of each treatment session. When my energy was low, having other people there kept my husband occupied and made the time fly.

- Offer to clean the survivor's house or even just the room they use the most.
- Gifts for the long hours of chemo:
  - o Small blanket and/or pillow, especially made by hand.
  - o Portable small craft project (if she's into that sort of thing).
  - o Home-made snack. Make it small and not messy to eat. Ask if she has any restrictions or preferences.
  - o Uplifting or funny card or a small book.
  - o "Mix tape" of relaxing or upbeat music or comedy shows in the form of a flash drive or CD.

~ 4 ~

CHEMO TREATMENT SIDE EFFECTS
Collateral Damage

"I have a nest in my panty," I remark as I exit the hotel bathroom. No worries, my girlfriend is used to hearing random thoughts from me. This knitting convention (yes, even this hobby has conventions) is a perfect respite for my husband and for me. I get away and focus on knitting instead of cancer, and Jim is assured that I am in the excellent care of a friend. This is important as it's just two weeks since the first chemo treatment, and the second one is in just a few days. The "nest," I explain, is my hair "down there" starting to fall out. What the oncology nurses didn't tell me is that the first hair to go may be my pubic hair. I focused on my "head" hair, but that isn't the first casualty, not in my case. Tears form as we laugh about this unexpected development. Laughing mixes with crying for this harbinger of yet undiscovered strings of body changes. Sure, the oncology nurses provide a list of common and not so common side effects for each drug in my chemical cocktail. But they can't predict how my body or the pathology of the cancer will react. So, my friend and I laugh – it's the only right response for us in the moment.

Aside from the anticipated hair loss, the remarkably unremarkable side effects of the first chemo treatment make the side effects from the second treatment even more unexpected—a two-day hangover. Sudden three-hour naps are now a part of my day. It's not that I get sleepy. It's an energy drain – something plucks the stopper out of the drain – and all the ability flows out of my muscles. Keeping my head upright is too demanding. Grasping my knitting needles is too strenuous for my finger muscles, much less remembering how to accomplish a simple stitch. As it turns out, fatigue is a side effect of the treatments. Going with the flow of my energy (or lack thereof) is something I need to make peace with for the duration. The "planner" and "doer" in me is frustrated, but much less wearisome if I remain flexible and listen to my body. There's a war raging in my body right now with several battle fronts. There are small, but aggressive battalions of cells that are out of control (cancer). My experienced, but somewhat outmaneuvered, immune system is trying to hold the home front. Chemo cavalry reinforcements have started to advance in waves and are engaging in many locations. Chemo is using maneuvers, however, that result in much collateral damage (side effects). The battle is expected to become less intense as chemo gains ground. But, for now, the war is at its height.

I'm not vomiting! Considering that nausea is a common side effect of almost all drugs I receive, this is great news. The strict regimen of anti-nausea meds is doing the trick. Just in case, I've been adding ginger ale to my diet after each chemo session. This shouldn't be a big deal, but I dislike the taste of ginger ale. A sister to the rescue! She sells Tastefully Simple® products, and she gave me their Cranberry Tangerine Drink Mixer. Mixing this with the ginger ale helps. One side effect of not experiencing the nausea side effect (are you still following me?) is that I may gain some weight during breast cancer treatment. I looked forward to losing a few pounds. But apparently it is common for breast cancer patients to gain 10 pounds during treatment. Diminished energy for exercise is one of many reasons cited. So, I am determined to get walks in every day – and I most often do. I'm able to do some gardening too – therapeutic. Starting a yoga class at Gilda's Club once a week may help too.

Gilda's Club is an affiliate of the Cancer Support Community. Gilda's is a non-profit organization providing support to anyone touched by cancer. I am fortunate to have a Gilda's Club near where I work. Their building looks like a small hotel from the outside. Each room is decorated like a living room in a house – not a formal one, but a lived-in one complete with afghans and well-placed tissue boxes. There is a kitchen, a large dining room, and a library with well-stocked shelves and comfy chairs. The books cover all types of cancer and related topics (nutrition, exercise, etc.). I became a member of Gilda's soon after diagnosis. Membership is free to anyone touched by cancer – the patient, family, and friends.

I join the weekly yoga class at Gilda's. It's quite informal, and the instructor is accommodating. I experienced two challenges in this first session. You see, I have difficulty with quickly distinguishing right from left. Sometimes I end up facing the opposite direction from everyone else in the class. At first, I felt apologetic, but this confusion became a source of smiles – sort of a running joke. One of my older sisters reminds me of what she tells the kindergarteners: hold up your thumb and pointer finger. If it forms the letter "L", it's your left hand. The other challenge is that I get nauseous in any pose where my head is lower than my stomach (think downward dog). I let the instructor know, and she helps me figure out alternate poses. The anti-nausea meds from the oncology clinic are no match for yoga.

Speaking of therapy, I decide that Jim needs some. Jim is exasperated with the limits of what he can do to help. He is typically male—he wants to fix things for me. However, he cannot fight this fight for me. But he can help me fight. And he is doing so already, in many important ways. Some therapy might do him some good though. I print off a copy of my latest mammogram, select the one with the best view of the tumor, and enlarge the picture.

I hand Jim the mammogram copies and the camera. "It's time you and this tumor have it out. Take whatever gun you want and have a 'conversation' with my cancer. Take photos if you want." You see, Jim is a retired police officer and the owner of a gun and archery store. He is comfortable around guns.

His forehead wrinkles, his eyes widen, then

"Come with me." I haven't seen him grin like this since my diagnosis.

I cross my arms. "No, this is between you and that tumor."

I'm not sure if this will help him cope, but it is worth a try. He selects a gun and is gone. I'm not sure how long – it needs to take as long as it must – and he walks back into the kitchen. Camera in one hand and papers looking like swiss cheese in the other. We both smile and hug. That's just the kind of therapy he needed.

The hair on my head is noticeably thinner with some bare patches now that I'm past the second chemo session. My eyebrows are getting scarce as well. Thankfully there is a "Look Good... Feel Better" class at Gilda's Club. This class is taught in the craft room. A large table is in the center with about a dozen chairs around. The walls are lined with cabinets and countertops with donated craft supplies of all kinds sorted into shelves and bins. I'm feeling that I'd much rather play with some yarn or fabric than with makeup.

The class is for cancer survivors and is sponsored by the American Cancer Society. I'm intimidated by the bag of product samples donated by major cosmetic companies. Except for some blue eye shadow back in the 1970s, I've never worn makeup, not even on my wedding day. The cosmetologist goes through the items in the bag. The woman next to me helps me pull out the items from my bag as they are called out as I don't even know what they look like. I'm open to learning, but my main goal is to understand how to draw eyebrows. I need to make them convincing enough for when I visit my mom. The cosmetologist asks for a volunteer to act as a model, and I raise my arm and smile. As she selects me, I breathe a sigh of relief, because I won't have to apply the makeup myself. First the cleanser, then toner and moisturizer. Concealer under the eyes is followed by foundation and powder all over my face. I feel spackled, but it looks OK when I look in the mirror. Time for color and definition with blusher, eyeshadow (oh good, something I know!), and eyeliner. I'm a focused learner as we are taught a paint-by-number method of drawing eyebrows. The finishing touches are mascara, lip liner, and lipstick. To my surprise, the result is pretty and not overdone. I'm even thinking my husband will recognize me when I get home. And I am just as sure that my makeup routine tomorrow will consist of drawing eyebrows. The rest seems to take too much time and money. My husband agrees that the result is OK – me, somewhat more defined – and he is also perfectly OK with not keeping up the practice.

Being around the breast cancer survivors in the class got me thinking about the term "survivor". Since I will now always have a risk of recurrence (however small the risk is reduced), "survivor" doesn't seem appropriate. Will I ever get past this and have survived? After doing a bit of reading in the Gilda's Club library, it seems I am already a cancer survivor. One becomes a survivor on the day of a cancer diagnosis. I get that, but I am still uncomfortable with the term since I am just beginning this fight.

These are some things I do every day now as a survivor:

- Spend time with God in prayer.
- Take anti-nausea pills for three days after each chemo treatment.
- Wash my face with a moisturizing cleanser and put on a gentle moisturizer.
- Draw on eyebrows, if I want to appear more "normal".
- Put on a head covering.
- Drink 80-90 ounces of liquid, not including anything containing caffeine.
- Eat five to six small meals to ward off nausea.
- Spend some time on the treadmill each morning if I have the energy.
- Avoid the sun since the drugs make me sun sensitive.

- Spend a little time on my CarePage blog.
- Massage cuticle cream onto my finger nails and toe nails.
- Swish and gargle with warm salt water to ward off mouth sores.
- Wear a soft cotton cap to bed.

And there is always more to learn on how to survive. Jim accompanies me to a lecture at Gilda's Club on treatment side effects. The speaker is an oncology nurse. She is well-informed and pleasant. This session also gives Jim and me a chance to meet others going through treatment – both survivors and their co-survivors. It may be a cliché that there is strength and hope in being with others who are going through similar experiences. But it is a cliché because it's true. Cancer can be a lonely journey – cells and drugs fighting a war inside your body. No one can pick up a weapon and jump into the battle. It feels good to link arms with others.

I'm in between treatments right now. My last treatment of these first two nasty drugs is next week. Jim decides it's time to get me farther away from home and engage in some retail therapy. His excuse is that he has nothing to wear at the Susan G. Komen Walk on Sunday. I suggest a pink boa and pompoms. No, that's not going to happen. He compromises and purchases a pink polo shirt. Pretty supportive for a retired cop who looks like a closely shaven Santa. Yes, my husband is my own personal Santa. And he presents me with a gift – a ribbon-shaped pendant with "survivor" engraved on one leg of the ribbon and a small diamond on the other. The necklace is a beautiful badge of honor.

At the starting line of the Susan G. Komen walk, I am nervous and grateful. Nervous about my ability to complete the 1.4-mile walk. That's such a short distance, but my body has been through so much that it seems longer. This late September day begins just above freezing. It will warm up later, so I am clothed in layers: jeans, long-sleeved shirt, Komen event shirt, bright blue windbreaker, pink hat, and a pink boa that I knitted. I buy pink gloves at the event, because I grabbed two left gloves from home. I really do have trouble with my right and left!

I am grateful to have the physical strength to participate in this walk. The day is brisk, but sunny. We walk along the Lake Michigan shore. The lake is a beautiful, sparkling, dark blue. I am brought-to-tears grateful for the people on my walking team: Eric for organizing the team, Jim for sporting the pink shirt with "cancer sucks" scrawled on the back in black marker and with his two middle fingers painted in pink nail polish (his way of giving cancer the finger), my son's fiancée, a couple of co-workers, and my aunt and uncle. Some drove hundreds of miles to support me in this walk. Their love leaves me teary and speechless. Hugs all around when we finish the walk.

Nine weeks into chemo treatment and today is the last session of these first two nasty drugs. My body will be allowed three weeks to recover, then the next two drugs will be administered every week. Today's treatment leaves me drained. I can't say how much of the exhaustion is mental and how much is physical. Being tired means slowing down. And slowing down means giving more attention. One thing I notice is that there is a tiny bit of fishing line (or something that looks like that) sticking out of the incision line of the port in my chest. This nib sometimes catches on my shirt. I ask the oncology nurse if this could be removed, or if my body will resolve this in time. "I could heat it up with a flame and burn it off," he says. He is joking – I think. He tries to hold it with a tweezer to see if it will pull out, but he can't get a good hold. "Will this be like when you pull a thread and the entire fabric unravels?" I ask. "No, your body just deflates," he deadpans. All the chemo nurses have a great sense of humor. That resonates with me and helps my attitude.

October brings a three-week break before I switch to a new set of chemo drugs. But first, the hangover from the first set. Menopause ended before my diagnosis, so I thought hot flashes were in my rear-view mirror. Not so. These drug-induced hot flashes are hotter than any I've experienced. I have so many during the night that I lose count. Feel hot. Flip off the covers. Feel sweaty. Feel cold. Grab for covers while keeping my eyes closed as I also snatch minutes of sleep. I remind myself *hot flashes are nothing*. Or maybe they are an indication of the heat of battle raging inside of me. *You need your rest. Just close your eyes and sleep.*

My jeans are too heavy. I can't believe I'm thinking that as I put on my new pair of jeans. I wore them yesterday. They are a bit thicker denim than my usual jeans, but it's getting cooler, so they seem appropriate. But those few extra ounces of denim seem too much to carry around. *I can't do it. Back in the closet you go. I'm wearing the broken-in jeans today.* Seems incredible that chemo fatigue is directing my fashion choices. Then again, I guess I've become something of a fashion maverick as I give in to whatever is comfortable.

Ouch! Please be OK. Yes, now I've started talking to my big toe. On one of my nightly bathroom trips (thanks to all of the fluids I need to drink), my big toe catches a glancing blow with the nightstand leg. *I'm so tired. I'll look at it in the morning.* By morning I see that all of the skin under the nail is black and blue, and the toe aches. My nails have become thin and brittle, and my skin is parched because of the chemo drugs. The oncology nurse advises me to ice the toe today, then apply heat tomorrow. I'll need to give up my short daily treadmill walk for a while and watch for signs of infection. The nail may give up its fragile hold altogether. I converse with my toenail – encouraging it to hold on. I've never lost a nail, and I really don't want to.

Ever since I started chemo, I've been swishing and gargling with warm salt water daily. This is to help avoid getting sores in my mouth. This risk comes from the way chemo indiscriminately affects all fast-growing cells in the body, and the mouth lining has these cells. But these cells can only take so much, and mine are giving in. I have an enormous sore on my bottom lip, and several developing inside my mouth. Now, before I eat or drink, I swish with a prescription numbing mouthwash. After eating, I brush my teeth and swish and gargle with warm salt water. This all makes me not want to eat or drink, but I continue because I know I need to keep my body in fighting condition. The numbing solution decreases the pain, but it also eliminates the ability to taste. Brushing after eating causes the sores to bleed and the salt stings. On top of that, I now have a list of foods to avoid courtesy of the mouth sores. For a vegetarian who likes food with a bit of spice, this list is a bummer. I am now to avoid citrus fruits, tomato sauce, spicy food, salty food, raw vegetables and rough food (crackers, for example).

As this hangover from the first set of drugs continues, it's mid-October and time to start the next set of drugs. Up to this point, treatments have been once every three weeks. They were nasty and were on the front lines of this fight, so that's as often as my body could endure. The new drugs will be administered once each week. They are the reinforcements in this battle. At this appointment, they draw blood to make sure my body has recovered enough in the past three weeks for assault once more. Since my body hasn't failed to bounce back each time in the past three months, I am optimistic. Dare I say confident? Jim is quite doubtful considering how rough the side effects have been of late. But Dr. A gives the thumbs up. He reminds us that the side effects of these next drugs are much the same, but in theory not as intense. And there are some possible new side effects. I dismiss the lengthy list and fix my focus on the end of chemo. If I stay well enough to make it through these last 12 treatments on schedule, my last one will be on January 3 – a good way to begin a year.

With Dr. A's blessing, a nurse shows us to the "party" room. That's what we've taken to calling the room at the back of the clinic. The "party" room is our usual spot, instead of one of the many treatment cubicles, because Jim and I are never alone. There's always at least one friend who shows up. This time there are several friends and family members to support us as we start the second leg of this quadrathlon. I'm starting to think of breast cancer treatment as a race – counting it down – what's left before the finish line. The first leg of the race is the first three months of chemo treatment. Now comes the second three months of chemo. Next is surgery, followed by radiation, and the finish line.

I give the nurse my "secret password" before she asks – my name and date of birth. In addition to the chemo drug, she will start the targeted therapy drug, Herceptin. The chemo drug, Taxol, has a high chance for a life-threatening reaction, so she gives a large dose of Benadryl through the port first. The nurse comments that I may feel a bit sleepy from the Benadryl. Almost at once I feel drugged – everything is in slow motion and in a syncopated rhythm. I'm relaxed, and words spill from my mouth before my brain can process or form them. I feel the muscles of my mouth and tongue forming words, then a short delay before I hear the sound. As others speak, I see their mouths moving, but there is a short delay before I hear them, then another delay before my brain understands. I'm living in the broadcast delay that television shows sometimes use to avoid airing something they shouldn't on live broadcasts. Once I become aware of what is happening, I think about not talking, but I'm so relaxed that I don't want to stop. I try to knit – something that I do at each treatment to keep my hands busy – but I can't seem to remember how to form even the simplest stitch. No knitting today. The intoxication lingers through most of the treatment. Jim and my friends and family are quite entertained. I am now looking forward to the remaining 11 chemo treatments for two reasons: each one puts me closer to the end of this breast cancer fight, and I get to have a legal high without a hangover. This is an unexpected treatment "benefit".

Although my big toe still looks awful, the sores in my mouth are all but gone. I'm back to swishing and gargling with saltwater daily to prevent future issues. Now I have insomnia as a new side effect.

How to deal with this? Nap when I need to but be watchful that I don't get my days and nights mixed up like some babies do.

As November begins, my immune system struggles. Despite precautions, I manage to catch a whopper of a cold. Jim says I sound like Darth Vader as I sleep. The cold is making me even more tired. I'm treating the cold by confining myself to the house, taking vitamin C, and using a neti pot (disgusting process, but it works). Since I don't have a fever, chemo treatment goes on as planned. The three hours of treatment seem longer today. I am tired – too tired to knit. We have a quick lunch with a friend who came to the treatment. I doze in the car on the way home, then take a nap relieved the cold is going away.

Or not. The next day my cold is worse. My immune system takes a beating each week with chemo. Fighting off a cold seems too much. I'm tired from insomnia. And I am missing my mom. Although she is about 20 miles away in an elder care facility, my visits with her are now rare. For her well-being, I cannot mention my illness. And I must disguise myself into familiarity for her – don a wig, paint on eyebrows, and wear a shirt that hides the port in my chest. This all feels too fake. And I feel unsure of what to discuss with her – the weather? Again, I remind myself to lean on my Father God and my circle of family and friends. I tear up. I love them all, and they love me. But I yearn for Mom.

After another month, my cold at long last seems almost gone. I am hopeful that I will not relapse again. I'm sending good, strong thoughts to my immune system – poor thing. My thoughts go to the upcoming mastectomy surgery about two months away. I have a list of questions written – homework done. And I'm confident the surgeon will answer them next month. I start to cry. I'm tired. I'm afraid of what removing my breast will feel like, look like, and how Jim will react to the change. How I will react to the change. This is overwhelming. I pray. God reminds me to stay in the present. He is in control. Focus on His love for me. Love and fear cannot occupy the same thought. Let love push fear out. Focus on the next thing and not beyond. This calms me. I remember something I read years ago: "The main thing is to keep the main thing the main thing" (*First Things First: To Live, to Love, to Learn, to Leave a Legacy* by Stephen Covey). I have nine chemo treatments to get through – that's the main thing right now.

The main thing I miss today are my nose hairs. You know, those little hairs inside your nostrils. I don't have any right now. I've lost all the hair on my body – everywhere. Those nose hairs acted like a furnace filter for air coming into my body. Now any bit of dust, fireplace smoke particles, and sweater fuzz become irritating. But the loss of hair has also brought me blessings. I have the look that is recognizable to those who know about cancer. Many girls and women have approached me – total strangers – at once bonded by shared experience. A teenage girl and I made eye contact in a restaurant. She simply said, "I don't mean to be rude, but are you surviving something?" I blurted the first words that came to mind – surprising myself. "Yes, I am!" and walked away smiling.

And just when I convince myself that I truly am surviving, Black Friday hits. The day after Thanksgiving is known for crowds of shoppers competing for deals. Not me. I have a cold again, so I will be even more housebound than usual. And I have a chemo treatment today. How to combat that grinchy feeling? Wear a grinchy hat! I located some fabric a while back with the Grinch character all over it. So today I wear my new Grinch head covering. The smiley reactions help get me out of my grinchy mood. I need to exit chemo with a positive attitude. This helps me through the several nights of insomnia that follow each treatment of these drugs. Knowing that the insomnia won't last forever helps. I read in bed at night and spend a lot of time conversing with God. He wants me to pour out my heart to Him – every thought. And I do. He's a great listener and he never sleeps.

Now I have another new side effect with these drugs, a rash on my cheeks that is a cross between a blush and acne. Sometimes it is worse and sometimes better without a discernible pattern. The doctor expects it to go away after treatment. For now, they suggest to continue to keep my face clean with mild soap and moisturized with a gentle lotion. The tips of my fingers sometimes tingle – neuropathy. But it's not so bad that it prevents me from knitting. And I've been knitting a lot at treatments and at home. The feeling of making progress and accomplishing something helps.

With five treatments left, my body is trying to fight back to a new normal. I have a thin crop of fine, downy white hairs on my head – as if cotton balls have walked across my head leaving wispy trails. This cottony hair feels just like the belly of a kitten. Is this the new normal for my hair? Dr. A tells me this hair will fall out as my new hair grows. No one can predict what color or texture my "permanent" hair will have. But I will never again think of hair as being "permanent."

A new month and a new cold. When I feel rid of a cold, another one starts. Thankfully the illness has never been bad enough to cancel a treatment. But the oncology staff does seem fixated on my weight at each treatment. Kind of irritating to focus on this, especially at the holidays. I'm expected to gain some weight with all the fluid they are pumping into me. Today they are concerned about a slight change from the last treatment. We determine that I weighed on a different scale today than the usual one. So, they weigh me again on that scale. *If they are going to interrogate my body's weight, I'm going to interrogate them on why they care so much about such a small change.* The nurse explains that my weight is one of the factors used when mixing the chemo drugs. And my weight change is enough this time to push me into the next "recipe." I suppose it's something like changing from an 8" x 4" loaf pan to a 9" x 5" pan when making bread. Well, that explains it, but it still doesn't make me want to get on the scale any quicker.

The big toe I bumped a while back is still black and blue, but the nail is holding on. Dr. A says it's just a matter of time before I lose the nail. Now the nail on the other big toe is loosening its grip. Merely a third of the nail is attached. I've added tea tree oil and bandaging my toes to my daily side effect regimen. This will help keep an infection from setting in. I need to gently file, not cut, my toenails. And I must be judicious in shoe choice – lots of toe room. I can still ride the stationary bicycle, but no more treadmill for a long while.

Nothing says Christmas like a new treatment side effect – spontaneous nose bleeds. This is a once every day or two event. The contributing factors are a lack of nose hairs, tender dry skin, and a cold off and on for the past two-plus months. My nose starts dripping blood. I sit and apply a cold compress. That seems to work. And as I get closer to the end of the year, an itchy rash develops on my hands and arms. This should be short-lived as treatment is almost done.

I'm not one to mark the passing of one year to the next, but this year is different. I'll be entering the new year with some big changes. The long tail of chemo treatment side effects will follow me into the new year (and beyond). I will bit by bit grow hair again in places that I want (goodbye wig) and places that I don't (hello to my new electric razor). The first week of the new year marks my last chemo treatment. And the first month of this new year will include a surgeon making significant changes to my body. As I enter this new year, I am a little scared, grateful, and excited to get a new year started.

I'm dressing up for my last chemo treatment – a plastic black top hat with "Happy New Year" in blinking lights. Once again, Jim and I have company at treatment. I am so thankful for that. Jim surprises me with a bouquet of white roses, one rose to mark each treatment. That's a lot of roses! There were no goodbyes at the oncology clinic because I will continue to come in once every three weeks to continue to have a targeted therapy drug administered through the port in my chest. This drug does battle with a protein that is on the surface of the cancer cell type I have. The side effects of this drug are fewer and less noticeable than what I've already experienced.

After this last chemo treatment, our group has lunch at a nearby Italian restaurant where 11 other people are waiting with balloons and a cake. Jim arranged a "No More Chemo" party. This is a great way to mark the end of the second leg of the quadrathlon. Surgery and radiation are left.

Where has six months of chemo treatment left me? Lingering collateral damage:

- No hair on my body, except for thin, downy hair on my head and under my arms.

- Thin and brittle nails with big toe nails that are loosely hanging on. Spoiler alert: Both of my big toe nails did in the end come off, then grew back in thicker and deformed. The podiatrist suggests coating the nails and the surrounding skin once each day with Vicks VapoRub. Yes, the ointment as a rule used to suppress coughs. He admits that it sounds odd, but it does help prevent issues from developing under the nail. Another spoiler alert: Years later, I decided to have both big toe nails removed forever because of ongoing toe nail issues.
- Parched skin.
- Itchy rash on most of my body.
- Numbness and tingling in my fingertips.
- Insomnia.
- Fatigue that is manageable by pacing myself.
- Chemo brain that is manageable with a good sense of humor and lots of sticky notes.

I now have four weeks to get my immune system strong enough to begin the third leg of my quadrathlon – surgery.

Helpful Strands ～
Chemotherapy Side Effects

Survivor

- If insomnia is an issue, do not give in to the notion that you may as well get out of bed and make use of the time and energy. Stay in bed and pass the time by reading, listening to music, praying, etc. Don't get your days and nights mixed up.
- Nap when you need to, but for no more than an hour. If you nap longer, you're more likely to have insomnia.
- Eat a small meal or snack every couple of hours to ward off nausea.
- Use a satin pillowcase to keep a nightcap from sliding around on your bald head.
- *After Breast Cancer: A Common-Sense Guide To Life After Treatment* is a book

containing candid and complete descriptions of what to expect after various treatments (chemo, surgery, radiation, targeted therapy drugs, hormone therapy drugs). I found the information complete and helpful. Be cautious about referring to this book, if you'd rather not receive the unvarnished truth.

- Wear moisture-wicking garments as they are more comfortable during hot flashes. Clothing designed for exercising works well.

- Participate in necessary and appropriate therapy for your body and soul. Ask your doctors and nurses for exercise suggestions based on your abilities and interests. Keep your mind active with reading, puzzles, or games. Nurture your spirit by staying active in practicing your faith. My husband took me on a trip to a mall for some retail therapy. Shopping for a few comfortable clothing items lifted my spirits.

- Get a cookbook that contains recipes targeting specific side effects. *Eating Well Through Cancer* and *The Cancer Survival Cookbook* both contain helpful recipes and eating tips based on the various treatment side effects.

- Helpful websites for nutritional advice are:

www.AICR.org (American Institute for Cancer Research) and www.CancerCenter.com/Community/Nutritional-Support (Cancer Treatment Centers of America).

- Use products to moisturize your skin that are gentle and fragrance-free. Avoid anti-aging products for now as they can be harsh. Lip balm can work well on cuticles.

- Use a gentle facial cleanser, instead of soap which can be drying.

- Gargle and rinse your mouth with warm salt water each evening to help keep mouth sores away.

- Wipes are more comfortable than toilet paper when you have no hair down there.

- Use packing tape to remove short, dying hairs from your scalp – like removing lint from a garment.

- Head coverings sewn from t-shirt material feel good on the scalp. Knitted caps of cotton or other natural fibers are less scratchy than man-made fibers. Buffs are easy and comfortable. A 36" square silk scarf folded into a double-layer triangle and tied at the back of the neck feels most like hair. The scarf is light, breathable, and moves in the breeze.

- Keep your perspective balanced. 2 Corinthians 4:16-18 states: "Therefore we don't faint, but though our outward man is decaying, yet our inward man is renewed day by day. For our light affliction, which is for the moment, works for us more and more exceedingly an eternal weight of glory, while we don't look at the things which are seen, but at the things which are not seen. For the things which are seen are temporal, but the things which are not seen are eternal."

- God desires to be your main co-survivor. Psalms 91:14-15 states: "He will call on me, and I will answer him. I will be with him in trouble. I will deliver him, and honor him."

Co-survivors

- Chemotherapy treatments can be months long and the side effects can be mentally and physically taxing. The gift of your presence is critical throughout this process. Distances can disappear through video calls. We even did a video call with my son during a treatment by putting our laptop in a chair. Encouraging and funny cards and phone calls are some ways to be present – even from far away.

- Give gas gift cards to the survivor to ease the financial burden of the numerous appointments.
- Give a cancer-related cookbook (*Eating Well Through Cancer* and *The Cancer Survival Cookbook* are two examples) as a gift along with a dish you've made. The cookbook may contain helpful tips to lessen side effects. Can't cook? Give a gift card for restaurant take-out. Your gift of food will help, especially if it can be easily frozen in case the ingredients cannot be eaten until after the current side effect is past.
- Shave your head in a sign of solidarity.
- Depending on your relationship with the survivor, accompanying them to therapy can be helpful to both of you, whether it be therapy to address the body or soul.

∼ 5 ∼

SURGERY
New Breast or Not

Less than two weeks after learning I have breast cancer, I meet with a plastic surgeon. After six months of chemotherapy, I will have a mastectomy. I've never been too focused on my body. A plastic surgeon's office is a place I never expected to visit. I promised myself decades ago that I would never change the body God designed for me – no plastic surgery, no hair dye, etc.

The nurse hands me a white terry robe as my husband and I follow her to the exam room. I take off all clothing from the waist up (something I will get used to doing each time I visit a medical person over the next year or so) and settle into the robe.

Dr. S enters and we talk about the possibilities for reconstructing a "new" breast after my natural one is removed. As much as a "new" breast will look much the same as my natural one when I have clothes on, it will not look the same when I'm naked. I will have to decide if I want a nipple formed and if I want an areola tattooed around the nipple. There would be a scar from the mastectomy surgery, and there would be a scar on my shoulder. The back of my left shoulder is where they would harvest muscle and tissue from, tunnel it around my left side under my skin to the front. This muscle and tissue would be used to help form the "new" breast. And there would be a bag of saline or gel silicone to make the formed breast the same size as my natural breast. All of this would result in something that looks OK, but the "new" breast won't have any sensation.

The process would take over a year in my case. And reconstruction would bring new risks. Rupture of the saline or gel silicone implant is a possibility. Capsular fibrosis (scarring around the implant) can result in hard lumps. During the four- to six-month process of expanding the tissue to accommodate the implant, I cannot have an MRI of the area. There are ongoing issues to consider as well. Harvesting the muscle from the shoulder can result in weakness in that shoulder. Having an implant means I would take an antibiotic before dental work. And it is recommended that the implant be switched out every 10 years.

I ask to see the before and after photos Dr. S mentions are available. "I'll have the nurse bring them in," and, since there are no more questions, Dr. S leaves me to get in touch with him when I have decided. The nurse returns with a binder. I open the binder as my husband slides his chair closer to me. The photos are in pairs. The photos are of women from the neck to their waist – a pair of torsos for each woman. The "before" photos reveal all manner of disfigured breasts – sometimes affecting one breast and sometimes both. "After" photos reveal breasts that are a bit "dented" with a small scar to some torsos with a large scar where a breast once existed. This is shocking. So many women. Not a result of war or famine. These torsos look fine and healthy, except for the breasts. I feel sick. This will be me. I look at the "after" photos for hope and for comfort. But I find none. Some "after" breasts look OK at a glance. But some have no nipples. Some have nipples, but no areola. Some have scars. Sure, this will do just fine when covered by clothing. But I will see myself – and my husband will see me – every day like this.

Even if I go through a year of reconstruction. This sure isn't the image I expected of a Hollywood boob job. Although I'm all for doing everything I need to, this seems way too much to go through for just a cosmetic result. As chemotherapy treatments begin, I decide to investigate the prosthesis option – the way less travelled.

Before long I see an advertisement that Gilda's Club is having an informational session on breast prostheses. Jim and I walk into the living room-like atmosphere at Gilda's Club. The large coffee table is covered with boxes and bags of products. Women are seated on chairs and couches set in an oval. The presenter is seated at the end of one of the couches. There is little talk, for the most part just nervous smiles. My husband is the lone male – I am the one person there who is accompanied by support. I didn't ask my husband to attend, he insisted. And I appreciate that so much. The presenter welcomes us and proceeds to explain about different types of breast prosthesis. As she does, she sometimes opens a box, cradles a prosthesis, points out a feature, then places it in the hands of the person next to her. We pass each "breast" with care around the circle. Some women take more time than others. I am amazed at how much these "breasts" look and feel like mine.

Mastectomy bras and swimsuits are passed around. I see that they have slits that the prosthesis gets slipped into. And the garments are pretty. They are much like what I wear now.

Although using a prosthesis means that my body is left disfigured and lopsided, I am drawn to the simplicity of this option. And I know I can have reconstruction any time in the future if I change my mind. Starting out with a noninvasive solution feels right. During the next six months of chemotherapy treatment, I investigate both reconstruction and prosthesis a bit more (see Helpful Strands at the end of this chapter for specific websites). I am grateful to have plenty of time to decide.

The time during chemo treatment passes slowly and quickly at the same time. About a month before the end of chemo, it's time to meet with the mastectomy surgeon again to prepare for the surgery. Jim is right next to me – as usual – as we stand at the hospital reception desk, my notebook of carefully researched questions clutched in my hand. I am fighting back tears as the perfunctory process takes a sudden turn. Dr. D is in emergency surgery (he is first a cardiac surgeon). My appointment must be rescheduled. My teary reaction takes me by surprise. Of course, emergency cardiac surgery takes priority over prepping for a breast removal. I guess I didn't realize how much I mentally prepared for getting answers concerning all that will be removed from my body. And I am eager to get a firm date for this third leg of the quadrathlon. And today is Friday. I take some deep breaths. There's no emergency here – it's just the weekend to wait.

The weekend is past, and it's December now. Jim and I enter Dr. D's exam room for the pre-surgery discussion. Once again, I clutch the notebook that's been with me from the start – full of questions, answers, and documenting my journey. Chemotherapy treatment ends the first Thursday in January, and my body will be given about three weeks for my immune system to recover. I remove the clinic cover-up from my torso (modesty has left the building) and ask Dr. D to show us where he expects to locate the incisions. He needs to make an opening to remove my left breast and an opening to remove most of the lymph nodes under my left arm. The surgery is considered a modified radical mastectomy with two-level resection. The breast is removed, but the underlying muscle is left. The two-level resection refers to the fact that Dr. D will remove most of my lymph nodes under the arm – more than 10 will be removed out of the 20-30 that most people have. He assures me that this is not a painful surgery – nothing close to the caesarean section for my son's birth or the rotator cuff surgery on my shoulder. I don't believe him. It doesn't seem possible that you can remove a breast and part of an arm without much pain. I let him know that I have decided to use a prosthesis. He needs to clean up after himself and leave me with OK-looking scars. He assures me he can do this, and that no plastic surgeon will need to mop up after him. I can be fitted for a prosthesis about four to six weeks after surgery when the swelling has gone down. The surgery itself will take about three hours, and I will be in the hospital three to five days. Simpler than I would have guessed.

Dr. D mentions that, since most of the lymph nodes in my left arm will be removed, there are precautions I will need to take the rest of my life. They seem overwhelming. How will I remember all of this? I make a list of my new restrictions and will post it in the kitchen.

- Wear gloves when gardening, handling garbage, washing dishes, or cleaning.
- Protect hand and arm from burns, including sunburns.
- Do not wear tight sleeves, elastic cuffs, watches, or rings on the affected arm. I make

an appointment to have my wedding ring resized for my right hand.

- Do not let anyone take blood pressure, draw blood, or give shots in the affected arm. I start looking for a medical alert bracelet.

- Do not carry a heavy purse, suitcase, grocery bag, or other heavy items with affected arm.

- No shoulder straps on the affected side.

- Keep skin well moisturized.

- Do not cut cuticles.

- Use an electric shaver, not a razor.

- Avoid insect bites.

- Avoid vigorous, repetitive activities. Build up duration and intensity of activity or exercise in a step by step fashion.

- Avoid extreme heat or cold for a prolonged time. For example, don't stay in a hot tub for more than 15 minutes.

We schedule the surgery for two months from now—January 31. I will have ace bandages wrapped around me at first. And I will have two drain tubes sticking out of my chest. Their job is to allow excess fluid to leave my body during the initial healing process. Each tube will be connected to a palm-sized soft plastic bulb. The fluid collects in the bulb, so the bulb must be emptied occasionally. I will need to keep a record of when I empty the bulb and how much fluid it held. When the flow decreases enough, the drains are removed. This normally takes about two weeks.

The two months till surgery pass quickly. There are pre-surgery tests to make sure my body is ready. And we have a Christmas party at one of my chemo treatments. The itchy rash covering my body (a side effect of one of the drugs) is clearing up just in time for the surgery. I have a visit with the oncologist the week before surgery. My blood tests show everything is back within normal ranges. Dr. A does a physical exam. He presses hard and can no longer feel the tumor in my breast. That's not to say that the chemo treatments got rid of all renegade cells, but there is no longer anything suspicious that can be felt. This is just where Dr. A hoped we would be by surgery time.

The day of surgery arrives. The nurse is looking for us as we get to the waiting room. There will be no waiting. We are 20 minutes late. In a little over an hour I am registered and prepped. Jim is nervous. Eric is with us too. He seems OK, but I'm not sure what he is thinking. I'm oddly at ease. An hour and a half after that, the surgery begins. The surgery takes just over an hour – much shorter than anticipated. The procedure goes as expected. The surgeon reports that he saw no physical evidence of cancer. He saw no abnormalities in the breast tissue or the removed lymph nodes. All the removed tissue will be examined to see if even microscopic evidence of cancer remains after six months of waging war with some nasty drugs. A week from now, I will have a post-op appointment where I will learn the results.

I am wheeled back to my room groggy but smiling at Jim and Eric so they know I am OK. I am lethargic and sleep most of the rest of the day. I am relieved that this third leg of the quadrathlon is done. Sure, I have some recovery to do, but I survived the surgery. Jim spends the night on a recliner next to my hospital bed. I tell him that I will be OK, but he insists. He hasn't left my side since treatment started. The way he loves and cares for me brings me to tears.

The next day, I am awakened before the sun by the sound of my name and a light touch on my arm. Dr. D has come to examine his handiwork. I wake Jim on the chair beside me while Dr. D turns on the light. Jim and I have been quite anxious about this moment. *What will my body look like? Will we both be OK with the decision not to have reconstruction?* Before either of us can figure out if we are ready for this, Dr. D has the bandaging off. My curiosity outweighs my fear. I look down at where my breast has always been. With the swelling that always accompanies surgery, there's a mini-breast – not even enough to require a bra. The 10-inch incision begins about where the nipple existed and ends in my armpit. The surgeon is pleased with how my body is responding. When Jim and I talk later about our initial reactions, we were both OK with how my left side looks. We both felt surprise in that moment about how much the change didn't bother us. I'm not sure why this part of the process went much easier for us than expected. Maybe all the sharing we've done about our concerns has helped.

Although my body is accepting the removal of a significant amount of tissue, my body is without doubt not OK with the anesthesia used in the surgery. After past surgeries, I have thrown up afterward in all cases from the anesthesia. I mentioned this to the anesthesiologist before the surgery. He assured me he would do what he could to make sure this experience is better. Instead of vomiting once or twice as with previous surgeries, I vomit when I have as much as one sip of water. So, the day after surgery is spent trying a variety of drugs through the IV to get me to stop vomiting. Nothing works, until a scopolamine patch is applied behind my ear. The patch works, and I am able to keep a liquid supper down.

The second day after surgery, I am able to eat breakfast and my pain is being controlled with Tylenol. I must admit that Dr. D is right – losing my breast and some tissue under my arm is not as painful as other surgeries. I feel better than I expected and am eager to get home. A hospital is no place to get rest. Someone is always wanting to take your vitals, give you meds, check to see if you need more meds, or just check on you. I should have brought a hotel "Do Not Disturb" sign. They mean well, but right now I just want to rest for a while. After we arrive home, I do just that. I spend the remainder of the day on the couch and go to bed early. I keep my left arm elevated whenever I sit or lay down – which is most of the time. This is to allow gravity to assist the remaining lymphatic system in my left arm. I have two drains: one under where my left breast existed and one near my left armpit. The drain tubes go from my body to the bulb-shaped containers (Jim calls them grenades as they are a similar size and shape) hanging in soft white cotton pouches from a Velcro belt around my waist. The nurses demonstrate how to care for and empty the drains. Jim decides to take care of that job. Emptying the drains happens several times each day, and I am glad for the help.

Four days post-surgery and I feel good. Any pain

I have is still controlled with Tylenol. The medical person who released me from the hospital (not Dr. D as he was busy with surgery) told me it will be OK to go for a stroll when I feel up for it. And today I feel up for a walk. Since it is January in Wisconsin, Jim and I head for a shopping mall and go for a short walk. Having energy and getting out with my husband feels good. I feel supported and safe in this adventure.

When we get home, that feeling of safety leaves. The drain tubes are leaking, so we call the surgeon's nurse. We describe what the fluid looks like, the volume, and that the source is where the drain tubes attach to my body. She asks about my activity level.

"Felt good, so we went for a short stroll in the mall."

"What! You just experienced major surgery. You need to sit or lie down most of the time. What made you think you should go for a walk?", she admonishes.

I feel like a scolded child. "The person who released me from the hospital said it would be OK."

She asks for his name and promises to have a conversation with him. I am relegated to the couch until my post-op appointment four days from now.

We don't leave the house for those four days. It

doesn't take long before I tire of lying on my back with my left arm propped up by pillows. The change in activity level is soon reflected in decreased fluid deposited in the "grenades" and hardly any fluid leaking where the tubes enter my body. There are a few arm exercises I am allowed to do, but they are gentle and don't seem to have a negative effect on the draining activity. I watch TV, read, use my laptop, and do one-handed counted cross-stitch.

The post-op appointment brings mixed news. The pathology results are in from the removed tissue. The tumor in the left breast is gone, except for residual DCIS (ductal carcinoma in situ) – precancer cells in the breast ducts that had not formed a tumor yet. Of the 13 lymph nodes removed, one still contained cancer. And a 1.5 mm tumor remained in the removed arm tissue. I am disappointed that six months of chemo did not destroy all of the cancer and that the cancer has gone beyond my lymph nodes. But Dr. D assures me that the chemo did a superb job. I am also hoping to get both drains out. They remove one, but the other must stay. There's still too much fluid coming out. How do they remove a drain? The nurse cuts the stitch holding the tube in place. She asks me to take a deep breath, then release little by little. As I do this, she pulls a foot-long tube out of my chest. My eyes widen as this magic trick appears from my chest. The process doesn't hurt, but is a creepy, weird feeling. I should be able to get the other drain out in a week.

As for next steps, radiation is certain and will begin in three to four weeks. This will allow my incision to heal enough to take the onslaught of rays. Dr. D mentions the possibility of more chemo but leaves that decision to the oncologist. Two weeks after the surgery, the other drain is removed, and I continue the infusion of the targeted therapy drug through my port. Surgery hasn't interrupted that schedule. I continue this targeted therapy once every three weeks. There's still eight months to go for that treatment. But, for now, there is a pause. Sometimes I don't see a doctor or nurse for an entire week. I feel a kind of new "normal" creeping back into my life. Good, I guess. I am a little uneasy though. I feel as though I am not fighting as hard against cancer at a time when I don't know how much that enemy has retreated.

Helpful Strands ∼
Surgery

Survivor

- The American Cancer Society has products to make the post-surgery experience more comfortable. I used their Surgical Drain Belt with Pockets. Instead of pinning the drains to clothes, the drains are in pouches on a soft, stretched belt under your clothes. It's best to have two – one for day wear and one to wear in the shower (when you can do showers). Their online store is at www.TLCDirect.org or you may request a catalog of their products supporting breast cancer patients throughout treatment.

- Keep a notebook dedicated to documenting questions for medical staff, their responses, your feelings, your physical symptoms, and your appointments. Date each entry you make.

- Don't wear a bra of any kind after surgery until the drains are all removed.

- Rest after surgery. Resist the temptation to do otherwise.

- If lymph nodes are removed, get a medical ID bracelet to caution against taking blood pressure or using needles on that arm. I found pretty, yet functional, bracelets at www. LaurensHope.com.

- Information on reconstruction and plastic surgery abounds. I found helpful information on breast prostheses and mastectomy bras at Amoena (www.Amoena.com) and Trulife Breastcare (www.Trulifebreastcare.com) among many others. Soma makes comfortable mastectomy bras, but they were not covered by my insurance.

- Consider thinking of the mastectomy scars as battle scars. As 1 Samuel 16:7 states: "But Yahweh said to Samuel, 'Don't look on his face, or on the height of his stature, because I have rejected him; for I don't see as man sees. For man looks at the outward appearance, but Yahweh looks at the heart."

Co-survivors

- Offer to care for and empty the drains.
- Make simple meals for the freezer before surgery. Soup works well. Freeze in single portions.
- Engage in reflective conversation. Let the survivor do most of the talking. Encourage the survivor to share. Don't judge or indicate that you know how the survivor feel—you don't. Each situation and each person is different.
- The survivor will be sitting around a lot. Offer to clean a room or do the laundry – any chore.

～ 6 ～

RADIATION
On the Rack With Ray

"Really? You're getting involved in my cancer treatment too?" I'm at my dentist now that chemotherapy treatments are done. Since I will be starting radiation soon, my dentist advises me to use a prescription toothpaste each evening. I should still use my usual toothpaste in the morning. Although the radiation rays are rather precisely targeted nowadays, there is a possibility of stray rays damaging the tissues in my mouth. The special toothpaste helps mitigate that by protecting and strengthening my teeth. And, since some of the effects of radiation are permanent, he suggests I make this a habit for the rest of my life. Spoiler alert: After a year, my dentist approves discontinuing the use of the prescription toothpaste as my mouth seems fine.

Time to begin the final leg of the quadrathlon – radiation. I'm eight months from my initial cancer diagnosis. My body has been beaten by treatments. But the end is in sight. I just want to get past these treatments and continue surviving cancer. Jim and I meet with the radiation oncologist. Dr. M is soft spoken and reassuring. She's comforting, but I feel like I need someone who is more like a soldier in this war against cancer. Dr. M explains the process and follows up with a page containing the details. Next week, I have an appointment for a CT simulation. The radiation staff will take information gathered in that process to program treatments customized to my body and situation. I will have 33 radiation treatments – one each day, except for Saturdays and Sundays. Meanwhile, I will continue to get a targeted therapy drug through the port in my chest at the oncology clinic. The port is on the right side and my left side will be irradiated, so there will be no conflict. Some days I will go to the oncology clinic, then head across town for radiation. Most days I will just have treatment at the radiation clinic.

I have radiation homework. I am to apply lotion to the area irradiated two times each day. But I am not to do this for the two hours before each treatment. Because of the aggressive nature of the cancer and the uncertainty of where it may have travelled, radiation will cover a large portion of my body. The area irradiated is my left side from the center of the front of my chest to the center of my back – from just under the jaw line of my neck to the bottom of my rib cage – skipping my lower left arm. They provide a plastic bottle of Unicare Moisturizing Lotion. Lindi Body Lotion and Aveeno Lotion for Sensitive Skin have a more pleasant smell, and are still approved by Dr. M, so I also use them. I should shave my left underarm right before the first treatment, as I won't be able to shave during the length of treatment. Picturing six-inch-long underarm hairs by the end of treatment, I am assured that radiation will retard hair growth. I am told that I won't be comfortable in a regular bra during the length of treatment, so I purchase a soft cotton leisure bra to combat gravity and give my remaining right breast a little support during this process. I have started doing left arm exercises to increase my range of motion post-surgery. As radiation treatment starts, the importance of range of motion becomes clear.

As with the other cancer treatments, there will be side effects from radiation. Fatigue from radiation treatment is likely to start after two or three weeks of treatment, and can last weeks, or even months, after treatment ends. Skin reaction of the irradiated area will start after about 10 sessions and will increase in severity until treatment ends. The skin issues should heal within a month after treatment ends. Dr. M explains that skin changes also help to confirm that treatment is making the expected impact. Lymphedema may start in my left arm. Lymphedema appears as swelling caused by fluid not being able to flow when the lymph system is damaged or blocked. Surgery removed most of the lymph nodes in my left armpit, compromising the lymph system, forcing the remaining lymph nodes to perform all of the work. Lymphedema is treatable, but not curable.

The day of the CT planning/simulation appointment arrives. Dr. M reminds me not to use deodorant for the duration of my treatments. She does approve continued use of the deodorant I use as it doesn't contain aluminum. I decide to forego deodorant and stay stinky for the duration to feel safer. Dr. M also suggests switching to a fragrance-free soap for sensitive skin. After this short conversation, I follow the radiation therapist to the CT room for the planning/simulation process.

I take everything off from the waist up and place

it on the chair inside the door. The radiation therapist grabs a small blue bean bag chair and places it at one end of a narrow metal table. I lie down on the narrow metal table with the top half of my body sinking into the bean bag. They position my left hand above my head with my left arm flat against the bean bag. Since I am less than a month post-surgery, the range of motion of my left arm (even with religious adherence to physical therapy exercises) has not given me the ability to get my arm in that position without significant pain. I hold this position as they shift parts of my body and the bean bag incrementally to obtain the perfect position radiation will require. After positional perfection is reached, a machine sucks the air out of the bean bag resulting in a solid blue mold. They will use this mold to efficiently position me for each treatment. A CT scan is done to obtain more data for planning where, how far, and degrees of strength for the rays. My heart is on the side to have treatment, so talk turns to the careful work to keep the rays away from my heart. This does nothing to ease my already rapid pulse. This is all so new to me. Another first for me are the two tattoos they apply to my chest. Each tattoo is a dark blue freckle. Dr. M weighs in wanting a bit more healing to happen from my surgery before radiation starts, so the plan is to begin radiation in a week or so. I'm anxious to start zapping any nasty cells that may have survived chemo and surgery.

A week later there is one more process, verification, to do before radiation begins. I am on "the rack" – the name I give to the metal table with my mold on it – for half an hour. My left arm is still tight. The muscles and incision feel painfully stretched. The bright spot is that this confirmation process checking that the computer, radiation machine, and I are ready for the first treatment takes longer than an actual treatment. As part of the verification, I receive my third freckle tattoo—this one on my right side. One issue could prevent radiation from starting on Thursday – the steri-strips on my incision. Despite scrubbing the incision every day in the shower, those steri-strips are all still attached to me. I am not to yank them off, but the strips must be gone before radiation. *Would they turn into crispy wonton strips if irradiated?* The radiation oncologist suggests slathering them with olive oil to help release their grip. When I get home, I marinate myself in EVOO, placing plastic wrap across my chest to protect my clothes. The next day in the shower, it is raining gooey steri-strips. Problem solved.

The day of my first treatment I walk by the black

and yellow radiation risk sign on the large, cream-colored door of the treatment room. The sign sends a little flutter of concern as the sign is reminiscent of the fallout shelter signs of my youth. The heavy door – a cross between a bank safe door and a large office door – gradually creaks closed behind the two radiation therapists and me. Along the opposite wall is a clothesline full of blue foam blobs of different shapes, each about two or three feet in diameter – the stiff bean bags. White cabinets and pieces of medical equipment line the wall to my right. A narrow stainless-steel table covered with a white sheet is in front of me. The first radiation session will take longer, because several chest x-rays will be done as a baseline. Then as treatment progresses x-rays will be taken and compared to check that my positioning is correct. I strip off everything from the waist up, while they locate my upper body mold from the clothesline. They place the mold on one end of the table. I lay down with care settling into the nooks and crannies of the mold. The post-surgery arm exercises are helping to make the arm positioning a tad less painful. The x-rays are quick. Time for the radiation treatment to begin.

The radiation therapists expertly move my mold and me into position, sliding me incrementally by pulling on the sheet under me, adjusting my arms, my head ever so slightly. The precision gives me confidence and makes me nervous at the same time. *Will I hear or feel anything? Will I be able to hold still enough? What happens if I move a little? Is it OK to breathe?* They plan to irradiate my left side from the center of my front to almost the center of my back, and from the bottom of my rib cage to my neck. The machine will move around me stopping at seven different angles to work around my heart and lungs. Each zap is 15-45 seconds long. I must lie downright still (but breathing is allowed) during these zaps for a total of around five minutes. The radiation therapists leave the room for the control panel in the adjacent room. They can see and hear me from the room next door, but that doesn't ease my nervousness as the thick, heavy door creaks gradually closed behind them. I focus on trying to slow down my breathing and stare at the colorful water scene on the ceiling straight above me where a white ceiling panel would be. I can hear music playing – my favorite radio station – from the corner to my right. *No, don't turn your head to look!* In between zaps, the radiation therapist steps in and adds or removes a thick plastic pad covering part of my chest. They call it a skin boost, and I make a mental note to ask the radiation oncologist in my weekly visit to explain this. I count each zap and am relieved after number seven. *Did I hear a buzzing sound each time she left the room?* The radiation oncologist comes back in and confirms that this session is done. I get my clothes back on and head for Jim in the waiting area. After chemo and surgery, it seems strange to have a cancer treatment that feels like nothing. At home, I spread lotion on the area they indicate was irradiated. Doesn't look any different to me. One down and 32 more to go.

During the treatments over the following two days, the strict routine of the process allows me time to consider what to think about as I lay on the "rack" each day. I feel as though I should use this time every day for something. So, I form a reflection routine for radiation. When I first lie down, I notice my left arm muscles clearly communicating how much they do not want this uncomfortable position. Next, I alternate between two thoughts. During each of the radiation zaps, I count which of the seven zaps I am getting, and I start counting in my head from one until that zap ends. Each zap has a different length. Between zaps I list what I am thankful for. Today I start with thanking God for the staff, the radiation machine, the knowledge given to people that made the machines, the knowledge that God is always with me, and I just keep going with whatever comes to mind. This approach helps me to remain still and helps relax those arm muscles that desire to twitch. Taking gentle care of my skin when applying lotion twice daily is also helping me relax and get more acquainted with my changed body.

With 29 radiation treatments left, the radiation oncologist checks my skin, reporting there are faint signs of a reaction to the treatment. This is good and is one way they know the approach is working as it should be. My skin doesn't look different to me. Maybe some of the skin is a touch pink. Or I may be imagining a change – wanting to see what the doctor sees.

A week into radiation treatments and just when I've adjusted to the routine, a treatment becomes problematic. The radiation therapist mentions she will be taking a couple of x-rays before we start and again after the last zap as a weekly check on positioning. I wriggle myself into the mold on the table as usual, and the therapists shift me around as usual until the alignment in the mold and with the tattoos is perfect. The first set of x-rays are taken. The therapists then leave the room to start radiation, and I listen for the familiar buzzing sound to indicate the first zap is being applied. No buzz. A therapist returns. She explains that there are over 200 tiny levers in the radiation machine that move to form the correct pattern for each of my zaps. This explains what I see in the machine when it applies zaps on my neck. The problem? One of the levers isn't moving into position for the first zap.

The radiation therapists invite a physicist to join us. As the machine is diagnosed, fixed, and rebooted, they ask me to maintain my uncomfortable pose so they will not have to go through repositioning me. Getting me into position and prepped normally takes longer than the seven zaps. We chat as the work is done on the machine. They thank me for my patience. *I am, of course, a patient, so I suppose patience is in my job description.* I ask if the machine has a name, other than 'linear accelerator'. They have never thought of naming the machine, but like the idea. They ask me to come up with a suggestion. I suggest "Ray". And Ray it is.

After the reboot, all goes well with the seven zaps. The radiation therapist comes back into the room. "All done," and she moves the table I'm on away from the machine. I don't sit up and slide off the table as usual. I don't move, continuing the uncomfortable position I've now held for 40 minutes. "Aren't we doing another set of x-rays?" Oops! She thanks me profusely for remembering, and says I am the best patient ever as she and the other therapist slide the table back into position. The second set of x-rays is done. By this time, I cannot move my left arm. The therapist gently shifts my arm out of the mold and back to my side. I get dressed little by little this time. My body aches and my left arm is useless for a while after the trauma of being in that position for that long.

About a week later, after treatment, the radiation therapists present me with a handmade crown – placing it on my stunted hair. The white paper crown is inscribed "You're a PERFECT patient!" in blue marker. A yellow star and pink dots complete the tiara. *I'm radiation royalty! After all that has been taken… I am now receiving.* A tear bubbles at the corner of my eye at this small, but exceptional, act. More good news—with 23 treatments left, I can without a doubt see that all the area being irradiated is pink – confirmation that the process is working as expected. Not so good news – all of this pink skin has started to itch. And I need to resist scratching. Can't afford breaking the skin and risking infection. I continue to use Unicare Moisturizing Lotion twice each day. And the radiation oncologist suggests adding Aquaphor Healing Ointment to a small spot on my mastectomy incision line that is more vulnerable to the radiation.

At 12 treatments to go, I can identify every square inch that's being irradiated. The skin is all crayon red and itches terribly. Cortisone is added to the set of lotions I apply twice each day. The cortisone takes a bit of the edge off the desire to itch.

Another radiation planning process is added before the final nine treatments. The process is needed to plan the radiation for the final five treatments. This is a special radiation boost applied to the mastectomy incision line. My irradiated skin is now a nasty brownish-red and looks dead. Gross. Desitin cream is added to my lotion set. The Desitin cream is applied in a thin layer at the evening lotion session after the other lotions are applied. *I've come full circle. My chest, back, and neck are now like a baby's diaper-rash butt.*

A couple of days later my skin starts to peel – starting in my arm pit. And I'm not sleeping well at night. All the irradiated skin is in some phase of discomfort all day, every day. Some areas move up the dial from discomfort to acutely painful and back to discomfort again. I don't enjoy showers right now, but they are necessary to keep my skin clean and free from infection. The twice-daily application of lotions and creams have become painful rituals, but the skin must be hydrated and tended. Radiation is affecting my energy level as well. Fatigue has set in. The doctor says the fatigue will lift two to six months after treatment ends.

After 28 treatments, I've made it to the final five—the boost treatments to the mastectomy surgical incision line. Since some of my irradiated skin has begun to weep because of the layers that continue to peel, the therapists take special care to protect the most damaged skin and focus on the thick incision skin. I now use Aquaphor Lotion on all the irradiated skin, instead of the Unicare or Lindi lotion. This lotion just feels better at this stage – creamy and cooling. The radiation oncologist gives me a small plastic jar of lidocaine-laced aloe vera gel to numb my skin as a last resort.

Today is the final radiation treatment. Tears stream down my face onto the blue mold as the final radiation treatment is administered. I try to hold in the sobs and lie still. I can't believe I've made it through nine months of chemo, surgery and radiation. Is it enough? Is the cancer gone? What happens now? Gratitude and uncertainty flow through me in emotional waves. As I dress, I am reminded to continue to lotion the skin twice daily for the next month. And there are actions I must take the rest of my life, because of the permanent effects of radiation. I must protect all the skin that has been irradiated by continuing to moisturize with lotion. This irradiated skin is now also more sun-sensitive. I must apply SPF 30 sunscreen every two hours when exposed to the sun.

Radiation footnote: I felt sort of a "full" feeling in the upper part of my left arm for many days toward the end of radiation treatment. This feeling is unlike anything I've ever felt – as if someone has replaced the tissue inside my arm with something of a bit more volume and much heavier. The feeling doesn't seem worse or better over time. With chemo, surgery, and radiation there have been so many parts of my body vying for attention that I decided not to deal with this potential arm issue. Out of curiosity, Jim measures the circumference of my left upper arm and compares to the same location on my right arm. Since I'm right handed, my right arm has always been a touch bigger than the left, but not enough to notice. Radiation has now made my left arm bigger than my right. A physical therapist confirms that I have lymphedema in my left arm. Lymphedema is fluid retention caused by a compromised lymphatic system. The therapist recommends I wear a compression sleeve and gauntlet on my left arm and hand to help my few remaining lymph nodes do their job.

The fitter for the compression sleeve is well-informed, helpful, and pleasant. She reports that the one color I can get is nude. "Nude" is darker than my pale skin. Having done my homework on websites such as Lymphedivas.com, I know colorful and pretty compression sleeves exist. I mention them, but she insists that insurance will not cover those. I inform her that I plan to DIY a sleeve with fabric markers if I need to start with a nude sleeve palette. My persistence pays off. She checks around and finds a company that sells sleeves in a wide variety of seasonal solid colors. And my insurance will cover them as they would a nude sleeve. She orders two sleeve/gauntlet sets in azure blue and lilac. Turns out that wearing the sleeve all day every day for six weeks stops the arm swelling from increasing. But it does not get my arm back to normal size. My left arm is bigger than the right, but not noticeably bigger. And the condition has stabilized. I can go without the compression sleeve for now.

After my final treatment, my husband throws me a radiation retirement party with friends at a local restaurant. Neon colored shirts and glow-in-the-dark necklaces make for a festive occasion. And I reflect on the past couple of months—physical and mental stages of radiation:

Stage	Skin-Condition	My Thoughts
1	Unchanged	"Is this stuff working?"
2	Pink	"I guess maybe I do see some change."
3	Red	"Wow! I can see every square inch that is being irradiated. And my skin is itchy."
4	Brownish Red	"This is gross. Will my skin survive this?"
5	Peeling, raw, weeping	"Ouch! I feel like a burn victim."
6	Thin, brown, peeling	"Interesting. This looks like shed skin from a snake."
7	Tender pink	"Sore, but maybe my skin will be OK again."
8	Tan	"My pale skin at last has that sun-kissed look – albeit in a weird pattern."

Now, a few days after the end of treatment, my skin is between stages six and seven. I believe my skin will one day be OK, and so will I.

Helpful Strands ~
Radiation

Survivor

- Check in with your dentist to see if you need to use a prescription toothpaste.
- Shave your underarms before the first treatment, and don't shave during treatment.
- Don't wear a regular bra during treatment. If anything, wear just a soft cotton leisure bra.
- If you have surgery before radiation, do range of motion arm exercises, to make getting into position for treatment more possible.
- Be dedicated and diligent in following the lotion schedule before, during, and after treatment. At various times, I used Unicare moisturizing, Lindi, Aveeno for sensitive skin, Aquaphor healing ointment, cortisone, Desitin cream, and lidocaine-laced aloe vera gel.
- Treatment may bring on fatigue. Accept it. The fatigue should go away after treatment.

- Decide what good, healthy thoughts you will focus on as you lie alone during treatment. I used the time to focus on people and things I am grateful for. This can be a lonely time. My faith in God assured me that I am not alone – God is in that room with me.

- Ask for and push for what you need. If I wore a compression sleeve, I wanted a somewhat pretty one. After investigation and pushing, I acquired one. Ask, or have someone ask on your behalf.

- Celebrate completions and victories somehow, however small. Just making it through a series of radiation treatments is cause for celebration as far as I'm concerned.

Co-survivors

- Offer to drive the survivor to radiation treatments. They are usually brief visits. Our 30-minute commute was longer than the treatment itself.

- Purchase a soft cotton shirt for the survivor that is loose fitting.

- Purchase a reusable water container for the

survivor as they need to hydrate, hydrate, hydrate.

- Ask before you hug someone undergoing radiation treatments as their skin may be hypersensitive.
- Bring food in individual portions for the freezer as preparing meals may be too arduous.

≈ 7 ≈

SUPPORT
Surprise

The diagnosis of cancer was a complete surprise for me – no family history and no risk factors. And the treatments brought new experiences, one right after another, for 16 months. But the biggest surprise of all—who came alongside to support me and who did not. This made for some encounters so wonderful that I cried at the thoughtfulness and tenderness. Other times were confusing and disappointing, leaving me sad and discouraged.

Job:

 I decided to be forthright with my manager and co-workers. Unless treatments were much easier than I expected (they were not), I planned to go on a leave from my job the day chemotherapy started and not return until active treatments were completed. I wanted to focus on fighting cancer – no distractions.

Our human resources staff followed family medical leave procedures for the first month, then turned the process over to a contracted disability company. I didn't always get prompt and completely accurate information from the human resources staff, but the responses were always compassionate. Their tone helped me be understanding and forgiving.

My co-workers conveyed their good wishes by sending cards and small gifts. A few coworkers even visited me at home several times. What an unexpected comfort.

My manager, a no-nonsense younger guy, didn't offer a good-bye, wish me well, or send a card during the eight months of my absence from work. When I returned, several days went by before he stopped by my cubicle. When he did, he focused on work. This left me feeling like an impersonal cog in the corporate wheel at a time when my body experienced assault in a deeply personal way. I'm not sure why he didn't offer an acknowledgement of my condition. Maybe he felt concerned about crossing a line. Maybe he was uncomfortable with breast cancer or with how I looked. I returned in the middle of radiation, so I wore layers to camouflage having one breast. My hair returned but was still unusually short. I never asked about his reaction, and he never explained.

Healthcare:

The doctors, nurses, and entire medical team were wonderful. They were experienced, helpful, pleasant, and often anticipated my medical questions and needs. They often dropped the ball in addressing my non-medical questions, not because they were reluctant to help. They simply did not know. Their attention and expertise for the most part did not include comfort of the body and soul. As I researched and explored solutions, I shared them with medical staff, so they would be better equipped for future patients.

Even when it came to durable medical equipment—what my insurance company called a breast prosthesis—my medical team offered no ideas. They could provide plenty of information on breast reconstruction surgery, but I did not choose that path. When it came to choosing a breast prosthesis and mastectomy bra, I felt as though I was the first person to ever ask. And how could that be true? The insurance company directed me to the one place they would cover a breast prosthesis and mastectomy bra. The elderly mastectomy fitter pulled out her most popular model of mastectomy bra—looked like a sleeveless straightjacket or maybe a breast girdle. Without a doubt not what I expected.

Next, I visited a charming store at the hospital where I received my second opinion – a place my insurance doesn't cover. The mastectomy fitter was closer to my age, experienced, and told me she could get bras that would look much like the ones I wore at the time – functional and pretty. However, she could not help me – even if I offered to pay outside of insurance. She apologized, but could not cross that insurance line. I just cried.

During chemo I researched online for prosthetics and bras on my own (see the chapter on Surgery). When it came time for measuring and fitting, I found the older woman no longer there. In her place, a woman younger than me. *Good. She will understand my need for a pretty bra.* Alas I knew more than she did. You see, she finished training for this job a few months before. So, I shared my research with her, and together we determined what to order. This left me insecure – feeling that I wrote my own prescription without any training.

Determining insurance coverage for prosthetics and mastectomy bras didn't go well. Every time I called the insurance company's 800 number, the representative informed me there was no limit to the number of covered purchases if I paid the co-pay percentage ("unlimited" was the word used every time). After I purchased an initial set, subsequent purchases were denied coverage. After months of phone calls, I discovered that there were in reality limits and what those rules were. The insurance staff answering the 800 calls were not given the information on the rules, so they were providing incorrect answers.

Friends:

Friends I saw often before the cancer diagnosis by and large didn't seem to go out of their way to change our interaction. Their support of me seemed not more or less than usual. I was OK with that but anticipated more. I didn't know what form that increase would take, but I desired frequent reminders that others were in my corner, holding me up, and circling the wagons to protect me. I expected more from close friends. And I felt as though I couldn't ask – or maybe that I shouldn't have to ask.

On the contrary, several friends I seldom saw or spoke with came alongside me in wonderfully unexpected and splendid ways (many of them shared in this book). The surprise of their creativity, humor, and love was an extraordinary gift of cancer. I will be forever grateful and attempt to emulate. Their gifts to me keep on giving through me.

Family:

My husband remained at my side every step of the cancer journey. At my diagnosis, he promised he would be there, and he sure delivered. He seldom left my side the entire length of treatment. Facing down cancer as a team deepened our friendship, marriage, and our love and respect for each other. My son loved and supported me in person when he could and from his home miles away – felt weird to receive his encouragement after decades of encouraging him. I am blessed to have a husband and son who are unconditionally in my corner. I know they are, but it was beautiful to witness this in action.

My family "corner" is crowded, as I have eight brothers and sisters. As the middle child, I seldom escaped family growing up. I expected these eight close relatives would rally around me. Timing allowed me to announce my cancer diagnosis to all my brothers and sisters at the same moment, in person. I saw surprise and sadness in their faces. What I felt were hugs. After that initial gathering, I felt as though they retreated from me for the most part. As time and treatments went on, many of them showed support in some way at times. But only infrequently, and I never felt encircled by the love and encouragement of family. This confused and frustrated me, leaving me sometimes sad and disappointed as treatment progressed.

About a third of the way through treatment, by way of reading and prayer, I gained some perspective on the variety of responses to my cancer diagnosis. Being restricted physically for a while, offered me plenty of time to reflect. I decided to view my journey from other viewpoints—what my diagnosis meant for my brothers and sisters. After contacting each of them, I found that their initial reactions to my diagnosis were different: shocked, scared, concerned, sad, wary, unfair, pitied me, and one even felt at once hopeful. Given that wide-ranging starting point, there should be no wonder that I would experience a range of interactions with them. My five sisters now have a medical history that includes breast cancer. Most of my brothers and sisters have daughters, and those nieces now have breast cancer in their family history. My three brothers are a manly group with a tendency to fix things. Now their sister has something they cannot fix. During treatment I looked different – a constant reminder of our fragile lives. As I considered this and other collateral damage from this cancer bomb to my family, I became more understanding and forgiving of their reactions. I always knew the differences of each member of my brother/sister tribe, and that my relationship with each is unique, and that's OK. I also know that ours is not a tribe that initiates group activities (reunions and fundraisers, for example). We each do our own thing. And in this cancer journey, each supported me (to a greater or lesser extent) in their own way.

Although support of family, friends, and others, was not at all what I expected, God is available to support me every step of the way. He is never more than a thought away, but He would not force Himself on me. Without God's support, I don't know how I would have made it through. That isn't to say I always felt His presence. On the contrary, I often focused on myself – just trying to figure out how to get through the immediate situation or trying to figure out why He allowed the pain or confusion or whatever else. What I do know is that when I focused more on God than myself, His peace came over me, my thoughts became clearer, and the 'why' didn't seem so important. I am grateful for each moment and trust Him for my future moments. I kept having to circle back and settle into the core of my faith – who God is to me, what He has already done for me, and what He has planned for me.

～ 8 ～

WHAT I KNOW NOW
Body and Soul

Moving through a cancer diagnosis and treatment taught me much more than I expected. Aside from learning about the medical aspects of the disease and treatments, I learned things about my family, my friends, and total strangers. I learned about me. And I am still learning. Here are 20 things I learned about my body and soul during my cancer journey:

1) Cancer treatment is the biggest physical challenge I've ever faced. Not the cancer itself – after all, I experienced no symptoms until treatment began. And the pain and discomfort were from the treatments, not the cancer itself. Part of the physical challenge is the pain of treatments and their side

effects, and the other part of the challenge is the length of time that my body experienced assault over and over. I understand that the treatments were timed to assault my body to its limit – allowing just enough time for the "normal" parts to recover, but not enough time for the cancer to regroup.

2) My body and this disease are a one-of-a-kind combination. There are high level ways to categorize breast cancer. But the pathology of my breast cancer, how the cancer gained its ground in my body, and how the cancer and my body reacted to treatment are unique to me. Throughout this journey, I learned much about the body's design, how it works, fights, and recovers. I pay more attention to my body. For example, I never considered my nose hairs. Losing them for a while during treatment made me appreciate them. A silly example maybe, but just so unexpected. I believe even more that the body's intricacy, complexity, and balance reveals a designer. I bow in awe of my Creator.

3) I no longer need to hide or protect my breasts. To this day, years after the end of primary cancer treatment, I often find my shoulders hunched forward. This protective posture seemed necessary after surgery and during radiation. But it seems to now be my default posture. I am focusing on getting

"the girls" out where they should be. Weekly yoga class is helping.

4) My husband believes I am beautiful – one breast or two – weird hair or bald. My husband and I both hoped for that as I started treatment. But this was new territory. How could we know? I didn't know if I would consider myself beautiful. We worked through this issue as individuals and together. We were honest and communicated about our concerns and fears before, during, and after changes. We spoke with those before us down this road – survivors and co-survivors. A key to this process is our knowledge that God designed me inside and out, and that I will always be beautiful to Him.

5) The tail of treatment is lengthy. Although some side effects were temporary, I have more physical changes for the rest of my life than I expected from the top of my head to the tips of my toes: thinner hair, a prosthesis standing in for a breast, an often-uncomfortable scar, a misshapen underarm, a bent fingernail, sun sensitive skin where radiation was applied, risk of lymphedema recurrence in my left arm, and misshapen toenails. And risk of cancer recurrence. I've experienced cancer once. Is the cancer still in me somewhere? Will another cancer develop?

6) Cancer creates losses, and these losses must be grieved to move forward. Losses occurred over and over as I moved through diagnosis and treatment. The initial loss of good health. Sudden financial changes. Emotional shock. Temporary changes due to treatment side effects – some changes becoming permanent. The loss of my breast. Co-survivors experiencing changes in how they see me change. Each person grieving in their own way and on a unique timeline. Allow for that. Accept that. And there's the knowledge that I will always be known as someone who experienced cancer – the loss of my "normal" life and the change to a "new normal".

7) Anchor to what is true for me. Throughout treatment and after, I continually discovered my truth. Sometimes different than the "typical" breast cancer survivor (if there is such a thing). I tied my mind to whatever stood true for me and acted based on that truth. My truth changed as I learned, but I always found an anchor.

8) Each day is once in a lifetime. Sometimes the day crawled during treatment. Sometimes the day flew past with appointment after appointment, then sleep. Fighting with time is futile. Embrace that day's flow. Appreciate each day for its uniqueness and what that day has to offer.

9) Fear is normal and can be helpful. Fear alerts us and helps us survive. Fear can motivate us to make changes. But feelings are not facts. Focusing on facts – what I knew as true – helped me reduce my fear. Focusing on what I am grateful for helped too. And the biggest fear killer for me is prayer – allowing my fears to tumble out to God, then reminding myself of who God is and what He does for me every day. Fear and faith cannot occupy the same space. Fear is a sign that I am doubting God's care and plan for me. Faith is reliance on who God is and His plan for me.

10) Don't assume—communicate. Co-survivors often assumed I was "fine" when there were no visible side effects. Clearly communicating my feelings and what I needed was key. This is something I didn't always do. Looking back, I appreciate what I learned about family and friends through their assumptions and their responses throughout diagnosis, treatment, and beyond.

11) Relationships change – or end. Cancer caused some of my relationships to drastically change or even end. Other relationships deepened. New relationships began with people I would have never met without being afflicted with cancer. Moving through these changes with grace at a time when so much is changing is difficult. In the end,

the relationships I have now are richer and sweeter because of the cancer journey.

12) Focus on the next right thing. In stressful situations (and the cancer journey is full of them), I recapture my footing by narrowing my focus to the next right thing to think or do. Scary times were often ahead, but I focused on just the next step. As Stephen Covey has stated in his book, *First Things First: To Live, to Love, to Learn, to Leave a Legacy*: "The main thing is to keep the main thing the main thing."

13) Be thankful. I had been a grateful person before cancer. The cancer journey has expanded this. I am thankful for the experiences I would never have had otherwise (well, maybe not all of the experiences). For the time shared with friends old and new. For the personal growth God is working through me. For my relationship with God. He never takes a break or gets tired of being with me.

14) Pay attention. Somewhere along the line of my cancer journey I found myself often being attentive to the moment. Maybe I tried to avoid pain that way. Maybe I was tired. I noticed details – the pattern on the ceiling. Noticed my breathing. Being deeply in the moment is something that helped calm me and is a practice I endeavor to continue.

15) Be clear. In the confusion of cancer some things became much clearer. I have an increased level of clarity in what I believe, what is important (and what is just not worth it), and how much I have yet to learn.

16) Keep forgiving. During the cancer journey, I forgave over and over again. I forgave myself, medical staff, family, friends – everyone. Extending forgiveness helped me keep my sanity. When frustrated, it helped to identify someone to forgive, and forgive them. Forgiveness has nothing to do with whether the person believes they need forgiveness, and forgiveness does not correct what has been done or said. Forgiveness is simply a letting go – releasing from my shoulders.

17) See yourself through the eyes of those who love you. With my changing physical appearance during treatment and the mental gymnastics I seemed to go through daily, I received encouraging comments from co-survivors daily. Graciously accepting compliments has never come naturally to me. Like many people, I am more critical of myself. I have learned more openness to incorporating how others see me. These words are gifts to receive – to take in. These are some of the wonderful word gifts I received from my co-survivors: amazing, hero,

beautiful spirit, blessed, brave, cool, incredible, strong, fighter, inspiration, positive, exceptional, awesome, disciplined, funny, superstar, rock star, super woman, and courageous. Thank you.

18) I am better and more capable than I knew. The cancer journey is so tough in so many ways. But I came out the other side. That's pretty incredible.

19) The end is sometimes just a milepost. As I crossed the end of the primary treatment finish line, I was relieved, exhausted, grateful, and uncertain. I'm done, but I'm also at the starting line of creating a "new" normal.

20) I am not the real driver of my life. I knew this before cancer, and reminding myself almost daily helped during my cancer journey. God is in control of my life. I believe God allows experiences in my life to shape me into the person I am to become or to help someone else. Therefore, I believe breast cancer is the right thing to happen in my life at the time that it did. Experiences may often seem unfair, but my life is in God's hands. He knows what is best for me. He can see the future, and how the experience will impact me and others. I am so limited in what I know and what I can see. I trust God. This faith enabled me to show up for treatments with a smile on my face (I am following God's plan for me). Faith threw me

into countless opportunities to explain the source of my courage (Answer? God). Faith made me fearless during many nights of treatment-induced insomnia (God never sleeps).

I shared a message at the party marking the end of my primary cancer treatment. I still believe these words.

"I thank God that I am able to be here today, and I thank God for family and friends. There is a special place in my heart for those who showed their support in so many ways during every step of my cancer experience. The love of God and the love you shared with me were (and still are) the cornerstones I am standing upon.

I named my cancer journey blog "Mercies in Disguise For Me" on faith that God would do a work in my life through breast cancer. Sixteen months later I can say that I have been forever changed for the better. And I pray that you have received something from this as well.

I want to share a bible verse that has come to me time and time again throughout the past 16 months. "Blessed be the God and Father of our Lord Jesus Christ, the Father of mercies and God of all comfort; who comforts us in all our affliction, that we may be able to comfort those who are in any affliction, through the comfort with which we ourselves are comforted by God."

2 Corinthians 1:3-4

I wish you comfort in body and soul.

Helpful Strands ∼
Websites and Books

These are resources I found most helpful.

Websites

- *American Cancer Society (www.cancer.org and www.TLCDirect.org)*
- *American Institute for Cancer Research (www. AICR.org)*
- *Amoena (www.Amoena.com)*
- *BreastCancer.org (www.BreastCancer.org)*
- *Cancer Support Community (www. CancerSupportCommunity.org)*
- *Cancer Treatment Centers of America (www. CancerCenter.com)*
- *CaringBridge (www.Caringbridge.org) as CarePages no longer exists*
- *ChemoExperts (www.ChemoExperts.com)*
- *Lauren's Hope Medical ID Jewelry (www. LaurensHope.com)*
- *Mayo Clinic (www.MayoClinic.org)*

- *MD Anderson Cancer Center (www. MDAnderson.org)*
- *National Cancer Institute (www.Cancer.gov)*
- *Susan G. Komen (ww5.Komen.org)*
- *Trulife Breastcare (www.Trulifebreastcare.com)*

Books

- *After Breast Cancer: A Common-Sense Guide to Life After Treatment by Hester Hill Schnipper*
- *Breast Cancer Husband: How to Help Your Wife (and Yourself) Through Diagnosis, Treatment, and Beyond by Marc Silver*
- *Dr. Susan Love's Breast Book by Susan M. Love, MD, MBA with Karen Lindsey*
- *Eating Well Through Cancer: Easy Recipes & Recommendations During & After Treatment by Holly Clegg, Gerald Miletello*
- *The Cancer Survival Cookbook by Donna L. Weihofen, RD, MS with Christina Marino, MD, MPH*
- *Bible in whatever version speaks to you.*

About the Author

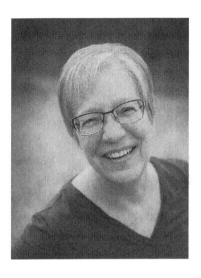

Rita Schunk is a Wisconsin native writing life's real stories. She grew up the middle child of a large farm family—straddling the line between peacemaker and instigator. After an extensive career in information technology, she continues her love of learning through investigating experiences of life, discovering what can be learned from these stories, and sharing the result. Rita lives with her husband and has a married son. Her passion for discovery compels her to a variety of handcrafting hobbies. She gifts most of her knitted creations to others – often to total strangers.

Made in the USA
Lexington, KY
22 September 2018